More Advance Prais
Neuroinfections

This is a useful, easy to read, "charming" book highlighting the com
and not-so-common infections of the nervous system, written by on
research neurovirology. The format of clinical vignettes immediately
asked and told what to do next. The key points in "What do you do
of the history, physical and neurological examination and support
neurophysiology, and imaging. A differential diagnosis is provide
approach. A list of suggested reading accompanies each vignette. Tr
such evidence is available, and when not, the reader is provided the a
rologist
useful ar
with a pa
nervous

—*Rob*

Dr. Gild
infection
bacterial
of inflan
typical c
with a su
practical
a wealth
mendabl
user-frie
previous
which m
achieved
includin
medical

—*I*
J

Thirty-fi
cal neurc
The cases
author d
tific data

—*Prof*

Dr. Gild
with a w
a case de
"Key Po
will be n
may not

This volu
"What d
ther read
concisely

What Do I Do Now?

SERIES CO-EDITORS-IN-CHIEF

Lawrence C. Newman, MD
Director of the Headache Institute
Department of Neurology
St. Luke's-Roosevelt Hospital Center
New York, NY

Morris Levin, MD
Professor of Neurology and Psychiatry
Geisel School of Medicine at Dartmouth
Hanover, NH

PREVIOUS VOLUMES IN THE SERIES

Neuroinfections

Don Gilden, MD
Louise Baum Endowed Chair
Department of Neurology
University of Colorado School of Medicine
Aurora, CO

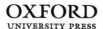
OXFORD
UNIVERSITY PRESS

OXFORD
UNIVERSITY PRESS

Oxford University Press is a department of the University of Oxford.
It furthers the University's objective of excellence in research, scholarship,
and education by publishing worldwide.

Oxford   New York
Auckland   Cape Town   Dar es Salaam   Hong Kong   Karachi
Kuala Lumpur   Madrid   Melbourne   Mexico City   Nairobi
New Delhi   Shanghai   Taipei   Toronto

With offices in
Argentina   Austria   Brazil   Chile   Czech Republic   France   Greece
Guatemala   Hungary   Italy   Japan   Poland   Portugal   Singapore
South Korea   Switzerland   Thailand   Turkey   Ukraine   Vietnam

Oxford is a registered trademark of Oxford University Press in the UK and certain other
countries.

Published in the United States of America by
Oxford University Press
198 Madison Avenue, New York, NY 10016

Library of Congress Cataloging-in-Publication Data
Gilden, Donald H.
Neuroinfections / Don Gilden.
p. ; cm.—(What do I do now?)
Includes bibliographical references and index.
ISBN 978-0-19-992663-3 (pbk. : alk. paper)
I. Title.   II. Series: What do I do now?
[DNLM: 1. Central Nervous System Infections—diagnosis—Case Reports.   2. Diagnosis,
Differential—Case Reports. WL 141]
LC Classification not assigned
616.8—dc23
2012038114

The science of medicine is a rapidly changing field. As new research and clinical experience broaden
our knowledge, changes in treatment and drug therapy occur. The author and publisher of this
work have checked with sources believed to be reliable in their efforts to provide information that
is accurate and complete, and in accordance with the standards accepted at the time of publication.
However, in light of the possibility of human error or changes in the practice of medicine, neither
the author, nor the publisher, nor any other party who has been involved in the preparation or
publication of this work warrants that the information contained herein is in every respect accurate
or complete. Readers are encouraged to confirm the information contained herein with other
reliable sources, and are strongly advised to check the product information sheet provided by the
pharmaceutical company for each drug they plan to administer.

9 8 7 6 5 4 3 2
Printed in the United States of America on acid-free paper

This book is dedicated to:

My dear wife Audrey, whose support and love have made my professional career possible and the rest of my life wonderful.

—DHG

Acknowledgments

I thank my colleagues in the Department of Neurology at the University of Colorado School of Medicine, each of whom reviewed 1 to 2 chapters in this volume and provided constructive criticism. Marina Hoffman provided an excellent editorial review of the entire book. Most important, I thank Lori DePriest for help organizing the chapters, figures, and references.

Don Gilden, MD

Preface

Increasing numbers of neurologic diseases are now treatable, particularly infectious and inflammatory disorders. As in all fields of medicine, rapid and accurate diagnosis is essential. In this installment of the "What Do I Do Now?" series, I have provided a user-friendly manual for clinicians dealing with CNS infectious and inflammatory diseases at both the in-patient and out-patient level. The volume is divided into 3 sections: (1) viral infections of the nervous system; (2) CNS diseases caused by bacteria, spirochetes, fungi, protozoans, and prions; and (3) CNS inflammatory disorders of unknown etiology. A unique aspect of the book is that every case is one in which I was involved either as a primary neurologist or in consultation. None of the cases is contrived; they are all real-time. I hope this volume will be a valuable resource for neurologists, internists, pediatricians, residents, fellows, and medical students. I have tried to make each case concise and precise, noting the salient features that lead to diagnosis. The ultimate goal of this book is to facilitate improved recognition and management of patients with infectious and inflammatory disorders of the nervous system. Key clinical points are provided at the end of each chapter. I have tried to provide optimal figures in many chapters to illustrate cardinal teaching points.

Don Gilden, MD
Denver, Colorado

Contents

Neurologic complications of Lyme disease are usually chronic and present as meningoencephalitis with cranial nerve palsies (the 7th nerve being most commonly affected and often bilaterally) as well as painful radiculitis. The skin rash of Lyme disease has a target appearance. Imaging abnormalities include meningeal enhancement as well as deep-seated periventricular lesions mimicking demyelinating disease. Confirmation of Lyme disease is provided by detection of antibody to *Borrelia burgdorferi* in serum and/or CSF.

CNS toxoplasmosis is the most common cause of cerebral abscess in patients with AIDS. Disease of the eye and brain often occur together.

Cysticercosis is the most common CNS parasite. Most cases in America are in immigrants from Mexico and Latin America. Tapeworm infection is acquired by eating undercooked pork and by ingestion of contaminated food prepared by a *Taenia solium* carrier with sticky tapeworm eggs under their fingernails. Seizures and headaches are the most common clinical features, although many patients with neurocysticercosis are asymptomatic. Cysts are readily seen on MRI or CT scan.

Jakob-Creutzfeldt disease is a rapidly progressive dementia associated with pyramidal and extrapyramidal signs, ataxia, and myoclonus. CSF is normal. MRI scanning is either normal or shows hyperintense deep-seated lesions, primarily in the basal ganglia and thalamus. How conventional Jakob-Creutzfeldt disease is acquired remains unknown although disease can also be transmitted by intimate contact from contaminated corneal transplants, electrodes, growth hormone, and dura mater grafts.

SECTION III   INFLAMMATORY DISEASE OF THE NERVOUS SYSTEM OF UNKNOWN ETIOLOGY

The clinical manifestations of acute disseminated encephalomyelitis (ADEM) are protean. MRI shows bilateral asymmetric white matter lesions that may enhance. Emphasis is placed on the need to treat ADEM with high-dose corticosteroids many weeks before tapering.

Viral Infections

1 Varicella Zoster Virus Vasculopathy

A 70-year-old man develops fatigue, anorexia, somnolence, confusion, and headache. The neurologic examination reveals an alert, oriented man who is imprecise and inconsistent in presenting his history. Muscle tone and strength and all sensory modalities are intact except for slight loss of vibratory sensation in the feet. DTRs are brisk, and both plantar responses are flexor. His gait is wide-based and unsteady. Brain MRI (Fig. 1-1) shows multiple foci of increased signal in white matter (top arrow) and gray matter (long arrow), particularly at gray-white matter junctions (short arrows). The CSF contains 25 WBCs, all mononuclear; a gram stain, stain for acid-fast bacilli, test for cryptococcal antigen, CSF culture, serologic test for syphilis, and cytologic examination for malignant cells are all negative; PCR for varicella zoster virus (VZV) DNA is negative. Other normal studies include: erythrocyte sedimentation rate; serum electrophoresis and complement; angiotensin-converting enzyme (ACE); tests for antinuclear antibodies; antibody to HIV; hepatitis B surface antigen and antibody; rheumatoid factor; antibodies to Ro, La, Sm, and RNP antigens; and anti-native DNA antibodies.

On day 6 of hospitalization, he develops right-sided ptosis and an internuclear ophthalmoplegia (INO). Brain MRI reveals a new right-sided parieto-occipital infarct and a small infarct in the right midbrain. The INO resolves by day 9, but left-sided weakness along with increasing lethargy and occasional myoclonic jerks develops from days 14 to 17. On the 18th hospital day, his left side is flaccid, and a right extensor plantar response is detected. On the 20th hospital day, meningeal and brain biopsies are normal. He is treated with prednisone, 80 mg daily, and his mental status and the left-sided signs improve. Prednisone is gradually decreased to 45 mg on the 37th hospital day, but 3 days later, his lethargy increases, he becomes confused, and prednisone is increased to 60 mg daily. Cerebral angiography reveals narrowing of the right anterior cerebral artery and slight narrowing of the right supraclinoid carotid artery extending into the proximal segment of the right middle cerebral artery. Cyclophosphamide, 100 mg daily, is started. In the next few weeks his mental status and left-sided weakness improve, and he becomes alert and oriented, although his left-sided signs persist. A few weeks later he develops increasing confusion and unsteadiness.

Multiple CSF examinations are performed. From days 4 to 23, there are 67, 60, 96, 51, and 34 WBCs/mm³, all mononuclear. Between days 6 and 13, there are 7,625 to 29,300 RBCs; on day 21, there are 491 RBCs. CSF protein varies from 143 to 202 mg percent between days 4 and 13 and is mildly elevated thereafter. CSF glucose levels are always normal. During the patient's 2nd month of hospitalization, analysis of CSF reveals the presence of anti-VZV IgG antibody, but not anti-HSV antibody.

What do you do now?

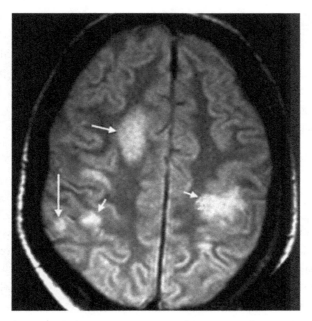

FIGURE 1-1 Varicella zoster virus vasculopathy. T2-weighted FLAIR brain MRI shows multiple foci of increased signal in white matter (top arrow) and gray matter (long arrow), particularly at gray-white matter junctions (short arrows).

Several clinical and laboratory features are noteworthy, including: (1) the waxing and waning clinical course; (2) the multifocal disease of the brain and brain stem as indicated by neurological examination and confirmed by brain MRI; (3) the narrowing in multiple large arteries revealed by angiography; and (4) a mononuclear CSF pleocytosis as well as very high numbers of RBCs at multiple times. Together, these clinical and laboratory features point to the diagnosis of an inflammatory/infectious vascular disease. The disorders to consider include the various systemic vasculitides that affect multiple organs, as well as sarcoidosis, syphilis, tuberculous (TB) and fungal infection of the CNS, and VZV multifocal vasculopathy.

The absence of systemic disease along with arteriographic evidence of large artery involvement reduces the likelihood of vasculitides such as Wegener's granulomatosis, lymphomatoid granulomatosis, polyarteritis nodosa, systemic lupus erythematosus, and sarcoidosis. While 15 percent of sarcoid occurs exclusively in the CNS, the likelihood of CNS sarcoid is further reduced by normal ACE levels. Meningovascular syphilis can be protracted, but a serological test for syphilis was negative. The negative acid-fast stain, test for Cryptococcal antigen and negative CSF culture helped to rule out chronic TB and fungal meningitis. While a persistent CSF pleocytosis is common in both TB and fungal meningitis, RBCs in the CSF are not usually seen in TB meningitis but are common in fungal meningitis. Importantly, two chronic CNS infectious diseases in which RBCs are often found in the CSF are the fungal meningitides and VZV vasculopathy.

In the context of the clinical, imaging (MRI and arteriogram), and CSF findings, the detection of anti-VZV IgG antibody in CSF, particularly in the absence of anti-HSV IgG, is decisive in the diagnosis of VZV vasculopathy. Detection of antibody to both of these human herpesviruses in CSF would have suggested the likelihood of a "bloody" tap. Overall, this is a typical case of chronic multifocal VZV vasculopathy. Imaging revealed both deep-seated and superficial infarction, and more lesions in white than in gray matter, including disease at gray-white matter junctions, a clue to diagnosis. While angiography revealed disease in multiple large arteries, MRI also showed deep-seated infarction in areas supplied by small arteries. Although the earliest descriptions of VZV granulomatous arteritis were primarily unifocal, VZV vasculopathy is more often multifocal. Also, disease more frequently involves both large and small arteries rather than only small arteries, while pure large-artery disease is seen least often.

Remember that viruses overall are small (about one-hundredth the size of an average bacterium) infectious agents that replicate only inside living cells and consist of DNA or RNA (but not both) and, in some cases, a lipid envelope that surrounds the protein coat before entry into a cell. In humans, viruses spread by person-to-person contact through food or water, coughing and sneezing, the fecal-oral route, sexual contact, and exposure to infected blood. VZV, one of eight human herpesviruses, is a ubiquitous highly neurotropic DNA virus. Initial (primary) infection usually leads to varicella (chickenpox), after which VZV becomes latent in cranial nerve ganglia, dorsal root ganglia, and autonomic ganglia along the entire neuraxis. Years later, as cell-mediated immunity to VZV declines with age or immunosuppression (as in organ transplant recipients and patients with cancer or AIDS), VZV can reactivate to produce zoster (shingles), pain and rash usually restricted to 1–3 dermatomes. Zoster is often complicated by chronic pain (postherpetic neuralgia), vasculopathy (TIAs and stroke), paralysis and incontinence (myelopathy), and loss of vision (retinitis). All of these neurological complications may develop in the absence of rash, as did VZV vasculopathy in this patient.

Standard treatment for VZV vasculopathy is intravenous acyclovir, the only antiviral agent approved for intravenous use, 10–15 mg/kg 3 times daily for 10–15 days. Because the inflammatory response may contribute to an immunopathology, our practice has been to administer prednisone, 1 mg/kg orally for 5 days (a taper is not necessary) along with antiviral agents. It remains unclear whether steroids confer any additional benefit to antiviral therapy. In HIV-infected individuals who develop VZV vasculopathy, additional treatment with oral antiviral agents (e.g., valacyclovir, 1 g 3 times daily for 1–2 months after discontinuation of intravenous acyclovir) is often needed. Indications for longer treatment include continued neurological symptoms, development of new MRI lesions, and/or an increasing CSF pleocytosis during intravenous treatment.

Unfortunately, the importance of the presence of anti-VZV IgG antibody in CSF in this patient was not realized, and he continued to deteriorate and died after nearly 1 year of illness. Not only did the patient not receive intravenous antiviral treatment, but was also likely further immunocompromised by repeated treatment with steroids and later with cyclophosphamide. Thus, anti-inflammatory and immunosuppressive agents can be a double-edged sword that initially reduces inflammation, but ultimately potentiates VZV infection leading to death.

Virological confirmation of VZV vasculopathy requires the detection of amplifiable VZV DNA in CSF, anti-VZV IgM in serum, or anti-VZV IgM or IgG in CSF. A recent analysis of 30 cases of virologically verified VZV vasculopathy revealed VZV DNA in CSF in 9 (30 percent) compared to anti-VZV IgG antibody in 28 (93 percent). In fact, the two patients with VZV vasculopathy who did not have detectable anti-VZV IgG antibody in the CSF were children with acute stroke whose CSF was examined before the development of an antibody response to virus. Although a positive PCR for VZV DNA in CSF is helpful, a negative PCR does not exclude the diagnosis; only negative results in both VZV PCR and anti-VZV IgG antibody tests in the CSF can reliably exclude the diagnosis of VZV vasculopathy.

As illustrated in this patient, many cases of VZV vasculopathy develop without any history of zoster rash. Equally important in the patient was the persistent CSF mononuclear pleocytosis with increased numbers of RBCs as well. While a mononuclear CSF pleocytosis characteristic of virus infection is encountered in most cases of VZV vasculopathy, increased numbers of neutrophils may also be seen. Elevated neutrophil counts are also found in VZV myelitis and brain stem encephalitis, since all the neurological disorders produced by VZV are typically chronic and active.

While VZV vasculopathy most often produces ischemic infarction, it may also produce hemorrhagic infarction, aneurysm, subarachnoid and cerebral hemorrhage, and dolichoectasia, and may be a cofactor with trauma in the development of arterial dissection. Table 1-1 summarizes the protean neurological manifestations of VZV vasculopathy.

Finally, the fact that not all patients with VZV vasculopathy have a history of zoster or varicella rash underscores the importance of testing all patients with unifocal or multifocal vasculopathy, as well as CNS angiitis of unknown etiology, for VZV DNA and anti-VZV IgG and IgM antibody in the CSF, since rapid and accurate diagnosis can lead to effective treatment of VZV vasculopathy.

TABLE 1-1   **Major Features of VZV Vasculopathy**

- uni- or multifocal
- infarction deep-seated > superficial
- white matter > gray matter
- gray-white matter junctions commonly affected
- large or small arteries, but more commonly both
- may cause spinal cord infarction
- rash not required for diagnosis
- CSF pleocytosis may include increased RBCs
- CSF pleocytosis absent in 1/3 of cases
- detection of VZV antibody superior to that of VZV DNA for diagnosis
- may cause aneurysm
- may present with subarachnoid hemorrhage
- may present with cerebral hemorrhage
- may present with carotid dissection
- may cause peripheral arterial disease
- all the above may occur in children after varicella

- VZV vasculopathy is often chronic and multifocal.
- The CSF pleocytosis in VZV vasculopathy is usually mononuclear, but because disease is often chronic, the CSF may contain increased numbers of neutrophils; increased RBC numbers may also be seen.
- The single best test to confirm the diagnosis of VZV vasculopathy is detection of anti-VZV antibody in CSF.
- Because not all patients with VZV vasculopathy have a history of zoster or varicella rash, the CSF of all patients with unifocal or multifocal vasculopathy, as well as CNS angiitis of unknown etiology, should be examined for VZV DNA and anti-VZV IgM and IgG antibody. Rapid and accurate diagnosis can lead to effective treatment of VZV vasculopathy.

Further Reading

Gilden DH, Kleinschmidt-DeMasters BK, Wellish M, Hedley-Whyte ET, Rentier B, Mahalingam R. Varicella zoster virus, a cause of waxing and waning vasculitis. NEJM case 5-1995 revisited. *Neurology* 47:1441-1446, 1996.

Nagel MA, Forghani B, Mahalingam R, Wellish MC, Cohrs RJ, Russman AN, Katzan I, Lin R, Gardner CJ, Gilden DH. The value of detecting anti-VZV IgG antibody in CSF to diagnose VZV vasculopathy. *Neurology* 68:1069-1073, 2007.

Gilden D, Cohrs RJ, Mahalingam R, Nagel MA. Varicella zoster virus vasculopathies: diverse clinical manifestations, laboratory features, pathogenesis and treatment. Lancet Neurol 8:231-240, 2009.

Aseptic Meningitis

A 23-year-old medical student develops headache, tinnitus of several days' duration, and stiff neck. A few days later, he experiences a disagreeable pungent odor that clears after a few minutes. That evening, he reexperiences the penetrating odor. He feels dizzy and attempts to speak, but finds it difficult to think clearly or express himself. His friend observes that he breathed deeply and rapidly while uttering incoherent words. He then has a major motor seizure. Upon hospitalization, his neck is stiff and Kernig and Brudzinski signs are positive. The CSF opening pressure is 310 mm H_2O. CSF is brownish, turbid, and contains small and large fat droplets. The CSF cell count is 24,800, 82 percent neutrophils. CSF protein is 7,200 mg percent and glucose is 25 mg percent. An MRI scan reveals a mass just above the sella turcica with a configuration characteristic of dermoid cyst (Fig. 2-1). A gram stain of the CSF is negative, as is CSF culture for bacteria and fungi.

What do you do now?

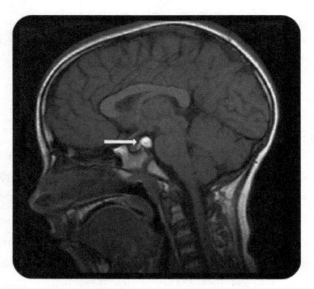

FIGURE 2-1 Intracranial dermoid cyst. Midline T1-hyperintense lesion, 11 mm in greatest dimension, and T2 hypointensity (not shown) is seen in the prepontine cistern and suprasellar regions (arrow). (From Indulkar S, Hsich GE. Spontaneous rupture of intracranial dermoid cyst in a child. *Neurology 77*(23): 2070; 2011. Reprinted with permission from Wolters Kluwer Health.)

The patient developed the clinical syndrome of acute meningitis. Historically, he developed an encephalopathy including seizures, and the neurological examination demonstrated the presence of meningeal irritation. The profound CSF pleocytosis, consisting primarily of neutrophils, along with a high protein and low CSF glucose confirmed the inflammatory nature of the underlying illness. In this setting, treatment with antibiotics must be initiated immediately while awaiting the results of CSF culture. Clues that this was not bacterial meningitis came from the brownish turbid CSF containing fat droplets and from the presence of a cystic mass seen on the MRI scan. The patient was diagnosed with chemical meningitis that was the result of rupture of the dermoid cyst. He was given high-dose dexamethasone, and his headache subsided within a few days. Repeat CSF exams continued to reveal high CSF pressure for more than a week, but eventually the CSF pressure returned to normal and the CSF became acellular; the last CSF protein on the 13th hospital day was 53 mg percent. After rupture of the dermoid cyst, only the posterior contour of the cystic mass was evident against the anterior aspect of the third ventricle. Craniotomy was not necessary.

Despite the presence of many thousand cells in CSF, predominantly neutrophils, and of hypoglycorrhachia, the CSF in chemical aseptic meningitis is sterile. The specific irritating substance in the cyst fluid is unknown. Aseptic meningitis occurs not only with dermoid cysts, but also with craniopharyngiomas and even in patients with glioblastoma multiforme.

Aseptic meningitis is most often caused by multiple DNA and RNA viruses. The most accurate estimate of the virus that produces meningitis is based on the time of year. Meningitis due to enteroviruses (Coxsackie and ECHO) is common in summer. Arthropod-borne viruses cause aseptic meningitis as well as encephalitis in late summer and fall. In winter, when mice carrying lymphocytic choriomeningitis (LCM) virus seek warmth and invade homes, humans develop acute LCM; also in winter, paramyxoviruses such as mumps and influenza cause meningitis. Both type-2 herpes simplex virus and varicella zoster virus (VZV) can cause aseptic meningitis at any time of year. In patients with aseptic meningitis and testicular pain, mumps virus is a likely cause. Similarly, aseptic meningitis in a woman with abdominal pain may be due to a mumps virus oophoritis; a pelvic examination may reveal exquisite ovarian tenderness. Abdominal pain in a patient with aseptic meningitis may also be due to mumps pancreatitis, and serum amylase may be elevated in these patients. Importantly, both LCM and mumps virus infection produces hundreds to thousands of cells in the CSF, and both LCM and mumps meningitis are associated with low glucose one-third of the time. VZV may also produce hypoglycorrhachia.

In addition to viruses, drugs can induce aseptic meningitis. The most common ones are nonsteroidal anti-inflammatory drugs (e.g., ibuprofen), antimicrobial drugs, monoclonal antibodies, vaccines, and intravenous immunoglobulins.

- Patients who present with acute meningitis must be treated immediately with antibiotics while awaiting the results of CSF cultures.
- Viruses are the most common cause of aseptic meningitis. Other causes are drugs and chemicals released as a result of rupture of a cyst or tumor in the brain.
- The etiologic agent in viral meningitis can best be determined by the time of year it occurred.
- When aseptic meningitis is caused by rupture of a cyst, the CSF is sterile and often contains many thousands of cells, predominately neutrophils, with hypoglycorrhachia and very high protein concentrations, thus mimicking bacterial meningitis.

Further Reading

Nettis E, Calogiuri G, Colanardi MC, Ferrannini A, Tursi A. Drug-induced aseptic meningitis. *Curr Drug Targets Immune Endocr Metabol Disord* 3:143–149, 2003.

Liu JK, Gottfried ON, Salzman KL, Schmidt RH, Couldwell WT. Ruptured intracranial dermoid cysts: clinical, radiographic, and surgical features. *Neurosurgery* 62:377–384, 2008.

3 Herpes Simplex Virus Encephalitis

A 45-year-old businessman from Chicago attending a convention in Denver is wandering the streets downtown. The police find him disheveled, confused, and belligerent, and jail him overnight on suspicion of alcohol or drug use. The next morning, he is sweating. His temperature is 101° F, and he is taken to the hospital for further evaluation. The neurological examination indicates irritability and incoherent dysarthric speech, although he attempts to be compliant. Cognition is highly impaired. He knows his name, but not his age or home address. He does not know the current US president and has trouble with simple arithmetic. He does not know how a car is like an airplane or how a shoe is like a shirt and cannot interpret simple proverbs. Visual fields are full to threat. Fundi are normal. He has a mild left hemiparesis. All DTR reflexes are brisk, and both plantar responses are extensor. A T2-weighted brain MRI scan reveals extensive involvement of both temporal lobes and the orbital surface of the frontal lobes with occipital lobe edema (Fig. 3-1). A CSF examination reveals an opening pressure of 260 mm H_2O, 50 RBCs, 38 WBCs (100 percent mononuclear);

CSF protein is 75 mg percent and glucose is 80 mg percent. A gram stain and acid-fast stain are performed on the CSF, and it is cultured for bacteria and fungi. The CSF is also sent for PCR for herpes simplex virus (HSV) DNA.

What do you do now?

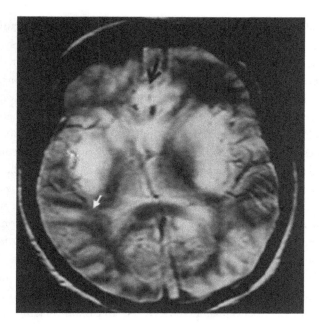

FIGURE 3-1 Herpes simplex virus encephalitis. T2-weighted MRI shows involvement of both temporal lobes that does not extend beyond the insular cortex (white arrow). Note involvement of the cingulate gyrus (black arrow). (Reproduced courtesy of Dr. Robert Grossman, Department of Radiology, University of Pennsylvania School of Medicine, PA.)

The patient's symptoms, fever, neurological signs, and CSF pleocytosis indicate encephalitis. MRI results showing involvement of the temporal lobes and orbital surface of the frontal lobes are characteristic of HSV-1 encephalitis and sufficient to warrant immediate treatment of the patient while awaiting PCR test results for HSV-1 DNA in CSF.

HSV-1, a neurotropic DNA virus, is one of eight human herpesviruses. After primary infection, usually in childhood, virus becomes latent in multiple cranial nerve ganglia. Reactivation is frequent and leads to recurrent sores around the mouth and nose (herpes labialis). Trauma (even biting the lip) and sunshine can trigger reactivation. Most HSV-1 encephalitis occurs after virus reactivates, although encephalitis can also develop during primary infection. Its occurrence is sporadic throughout the year. Herpes labialis is not usually present.

The clinical features of HSV-1 encephalitis are a consequence of virus replication and accompanying inflammation in the medial temporal lobe and orbital surface of the frontal lobe. In addition to fever, the neurological symptoms and signs are protean and include any combination of headache, irritability, and lethargy, as well as confusion, seizures (major motor, complex partial, focal, and even absence attacks), aphasia (when the dominant temporal lobe is involved), and focal motor or sensory deficit. Extensive hemorrhagic necrosis and temporal lobe edema may progress to uncal herniation. Because HSV-1 becomes latent and periodically reactivates to produce recurrent herpes labialis, there is the misconception that HSV-1 encephalitis is protracted or chronic. While survivors of HSV-1 encephalitis may have a permanent seizure disorder, memory loss, aphasia, or motor deficit, the onset of neurologic disease is usually acute, as in other viral encephalitides, and early treatment is crucial to a favorable outcome. Of all the viral encephalitides, HSV-1 encephalitis is most amenable to diagnosis by laboratory tests, the most important of which is PCR detection of HSV-1 DNA in CSF. PCR, which is both sensitive and specific, has become the gold standard and obviates the need for brain biopsy in suspected cases of HSV-1 encephalitis. CSF examination, electroencephalography (EEG) and brain imaging all have a role in diagnosis and should be performed whenever HSV-1 encephalitis is suspected. The CSF is usually abnormal in HSV-1 encephalitis. CSF opening pressure may be normal or very high if there is brain swelling and impending temporal lobe herniation. CSF examination should be performed in the first few days of illness, before significant brain swelling, to lessen concern over potential herniation after lumbar puncture. Approximately 90 percent of patients have CSF pleocytosis, although its absence does not rule out HSV-1 encephalitis. CSF cells range from 4 to 755/mm³. The predominant cell type is mononuclear. Unlike most other viral encephalitides, the CSF in HSV-1 encephalitis is often xanthochromic and contains RBCs, likely reflecting the hemorrhagic nature of brain lesions. Instead of attributing the presence of RBCs in CSF to a "bloody tap," the astute clinician may use their occurrence to support the presumptive diagnosis of HSV-1 encephalitis. The CSF protein is elevated in most cases. Because antibodies to HSV-1 in CSF are not usually detected until 2 or more weeks after onset of disease, the practical value of their presence lies more in retrospective diagnosis. Rarely, hypoglycorrhachia occurs. Although HSV-1 has been isolated from brain biopsy or even autopsy material, the isolation of HSV-1 from CSF during acute disease is exceptional for no known reason.

EEG and imaging studies may demonstrate features highly suggestive of HSV-1 encephalitis. The EEG shows background disorganization with generalized and focal slowing, predominantly over the involved temporal region. Within days, widespread, periodic, stereotyped sharp-and-slow-wave transients may develop, usually at regular intervals of 2–3 seconds (Fig. 3-2). Bilateral periodic transients are seen if both sides of the brain are involved. While bilateral periodic transients may also be seen in other CNS disorders (tumor, abscess, subacute sclerosing panencephalitis, infarct, anoxia), their presence in the clinical setting of fever and rapidly progressive neurologic disease is strong presumptive evidence of HSV-1 encephalitis.

Brain CT scanning shows hypodense lesions involving the medial temporal regions. Before edema is extensive, an important early diagnostic clue is a sharp transition from the hypodense temporal lesion to the relatively hyperdense lateral basal ganglia. Edema and mass effect occur in 80 percent of cases, and contrast enhancement is common. MRI reveals a decrease in T1 and increase in T2 signal, and the abnormality includes a larger area of brain than is usually seen by CT scanning. Unlike CT scanning, MRI of the temporal lobes is not subject to artifact from the petrous and sphenoid bones, which often obscure the temporal fossa. A comparison of CT and MRI in HSV-1 encephalitis showed that temporal lobe inflammation was obvious on MRI days before CT changes. Diffusion-weighted imaging abnormalities may antedate and be more extensive than abnormalities seen on T2 and FLAIR sequences. Remember that the MRI in HSV-1 encephalitis may be normal during the first 2 days of illness. In that case, a repeat study is indicated if HSV-1 encephalitis is suspected.

Before the use of acyclovir, the mortality in untreated cases of HSV-1 encephalitis was 60–70 percent. Treatment with intravenous acyclovir has reduced the mortality to slightly less than 30 percent. Early treatment (before brain swelling and coma ensue) is associated with a more favorable

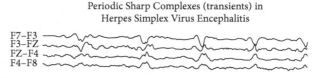

Periodic Sharp Complexes (transients) in
Herpes Simplex Virus Encephalitis

FIGURE 3-2 EEG shows bilateral periodic sharp transients.

outcome. Acyclovir is generally safe, although mild hematologic, hepatic, and renal function abnormalities have been reported.

While there are no controlled studies on the prophylactic use of steroids in HSV-1 encephalitis, I administer steroids, usually oral prednisone, 1 mg/kg body weight for 5 days (no taper is necessary) to control brain swelling. I have seen multiple cases of "relapse" of HSV-1 encephalitis in which the patient was diagnosed and treated early with intravenous acyclovir and improved for a few days but then deteriorated due to brain swelling. The benefit of a short course of steroids to treat cerebral edema and impending herniation concurrent with intravenous acyclovir therapy and intracranial pressure monitoring when necessary outweighs the small risk of potentiating HSV-1 infection. Finally, anticonvulsants are used to treat seizures.

The patient presented herein did have a positive CSF PCR for HSV DNA and responded well to treatment with intravenous acyclovir and prednisone. Transient sharp waves did not develop on EEG.

Note that HSV-2 (the cause of genital herpes) also causes encephalitis, with most, but not all, cases developing in infants and children. There are more similarities than differences in the clinical features of HSV-1 and HSV-2 encephalitis, although MRI in the latter often reveals lesions in sites beyond the temporal lobe. Treatment is the same as for HSV-1 encephalitis.

KEY POINTS TO REMEMBER

- Because the neurological symptoms and signs of HSV-1 encephalitis are protean and may include any combination of acute headache, behavioral and/or mental status changes, aphasia, seizures or focal deficit, the clinician must have a high index of suspicion and begin treatment with intravenous acyclovir while awaiting results of imaging, EEG, routine CSF studies and PCR on CSF for HSV DNA.
- The clinical features of HSV-1 encephalitis are a consequence of virus replication and accompanying inflammation in the medial temporal lobe and orbital surface of the frontal lobe. No other virus produces the imaging changes seen in HSV-1 encephalitis.

- While not specific for HSV-1 encephalitis, the presence of RBCs in CSF and periodic transient sharp waves on EEG support the diagnosis.
- Death from HSV-1 encephalitis is usually due to uncal herniation from cerebral edema. The benefit of a short course of steroids to treat cerebral edema and impending herniation outweigh the small risk of potentiating HSV infection.

Further Reading

Gilden DH. Herpesvirus infections of the central nervous system. In: *Infectious Diseases of the Nervous System* (Martin JB, Tyler KL, eds). Philadelphia, PA: Davis, Chap 4, 76–102, 1993.

Lakeman FD, Whitley RJ, and the National Institute of Allergy and Infectious Diseases Collaborative Antiviral Study Group. Diagnosis of herpes simplex encephalitis: application of polymerase chain reaction to cerebrospinal fluid from brain-biopsied patients and correlation with disease. *J Infect Dis 171*:857–863, 1995.

Gilden DH. Acute viral infections of the nervous system. In: *Scientific American Medicine* (Dale DC, Federman DD, eds). New York: Scientific American, Chap 16, 1–9, 1997.

4 HIV Encephalitis

A 38-year-old homosexual man developed acute headache, fever, and stiff neck. Except for nuchal rigidity, there were no other neurological signs. A brain MRI scan was normal. The CSF contained 42 WBCs, all mononuclear, and CSF protein was 70 mg percent and CSF glucose was normal. No antibody to HIV was detected in serum or CSF. In the next 2 years, the patient becomes forgetful, exhibiting impaired concentration and complains of difficulty reading, leg weakness, and unsteadiness on walking. His fine-motor movements become slow and imprecise, and his facial expression becomes less animated. He begins to withdraw socially, with a softening voice and loss of sexual drive. Six months after he develops neurological disease, a repeat test for serum antibody to HIV is positive. A CBC, chemistry profile, thyroid function studies, and vitamin B12 level are all normal. An MRI scan 1 year after the onset of cognitive and motor problems shows cortical atrophy and symmetric attenuation of white matter (Fig. 4-1). Another CSF exam reveals 25 WBCs, all mononuclear; CSF protein is 85 mg percent and glucose is normal; serology is negative. Acid-fast stain on CSF, culture for bacteria and fungi, and test for cryptococcal antigen are negative. PCR of CSF reveals a high HIV RNA load and is negative for varicella zoster virus (VZV) and cytomegalovirus (CMV) DNA.

What do you do now?

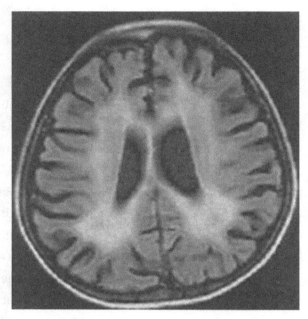

FIGURE 4-1 HIV encephalitis. MRI reveals cortical atrophy and diffuse high T2-FLAIR signal in the white matter.

The initial approach to diagnosis in a cognitively impaired HIV+ patient, with or without motor deficit, is exclusion of other treatable causes of dementia. The first analyses should be for hematology and chemistry profile, thyroid function, and vitamin B12 levels. The CSF should be examined not only for HIV load, but also to rule out opportunistic infections.

Focal disease seen on MRI might indicate toxoplasmosis, JC virus, or VZV infection, neurosyphilis, fungal infection, or lymphoma. Periventricular enhancement on MRI suggests CMV encephalitis and the need for a CSF PCR for CMV DNA. Meningeal enhancement on MRI is common in cryptococcal and tuberculous meningitis.

The atrophy and white matter attenuation seen on MRI are classic features of HIV encephalitis. The presence of acute viral meningitis a few weeks after primary HIV infection and before seroconversion is not unusual in patients who develop HIV encephalitis. Any likelihood of a superimposed opportunistic infection commonly seen in HIV+ and AIDS patients was minimized by the normal studies listed above. Further confirmation of pure HIV encephalitis was provided by a high HIV RNA load in CSF.

In the past, terms such as "HIV dementia" and "AIDS-dementia complex" have been used. Although neurons do not appear to be the primary cells infected by HIV in brain, virus is nevertheless present, and thus this disorder should be called HIV encephalitis. Prompt therapy should be instituted with HAART.

KEY POINTS TO REMEMBER

- HIV encephalitis is slowly progressive.
- MRI changes are characterized by cortical atrophy and white matter attenuation.
- In HIV+ individuals or AIDS patients who develop neurological disease, opportunistic infection (syphilis, toxoplasmosis, VZV, CMV, tuberculous, fungal infection) and lymphoma must be ruled out.

Further Reading

Avison M, Berger, JR, McArthur JC, Nath A. HIV meningitis and dementia. In: *Clinical Neurovirology* (Nath A, Berger JR, eds). New York: Marcel Dekker, Chap 11, 251-276, 2003.

Nath A. Human immunodeficiency virus infections. In: *Current Therapy in Neurologic Disease*, 7th edition (Johnson RT, Griffin JW, McArthur JC, eds). St. Louis, MO: Mosby Elsevier, Chap 6, 144-148, 2006.

Ramsay Hunt Syndrome

A 60-year-old man develops a dull nagging pain over his left mastoid area and in the left ear. A few hours later, he notes saliva dripping from his mouth. In the mirror, his face is distorted and pulled to one side. The left eye looks stonily as he tries to close the eyelid. When brushing his teeth, he cannot spit straight into the sink. At dinner that night, food that lodges between his cheek and teeth has to be pulled out with his index finger. Neurological examination in the emergency room that evening reveals paralysis of muscles supplied by the left facial nerve. On the left side, he cannot wrinkle his forehead, frown, close his eye, inflate his cheek, sneer, or whistle. The left eye is reddened from exposure to dust. A few erythematous vesicular lesions are seen in the left ear.

What do you do now?

The combination of peripheral facial weakness and ipsilateral zoster oticus (rash on the ear) constitutes the Ramsay Hunt syndrome and is due to reactivation of varicella zoster virus (VZV) from the geniculate (facial nerve) ganglion. In this syndrome, rash occurs not only in the ear, but also on the palate or anterior two-thirds of the tongue (Fig. 5-1),

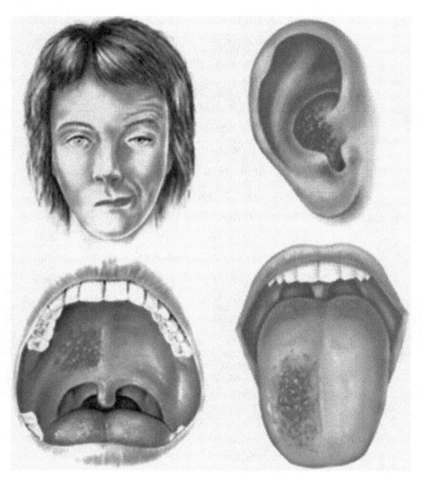

FIGURE 5-1 The Ramsay Hunt syndrome. The patient's right peripheral facial weakness, manifest by a widened palpebral fissure and decreased forehead wrinkling and smile, can be associated with rash in the ipsilateral ear, on the hard palate or on the anterior two-thirds of the tongue. (Reproduced from *J Neurol Neurosurg Psychiatry 71*:149-154, 2001, with permission from BMJ Publishing Group Ltd.)

sites that are innervated by the facial nerve. Although this patient did not experience dizziness, vertigo, or hearing loss indicative of 8th nerve involvement, those symptoms are common in the Ramsay Hunt syndrome due to the close proximity of the geniculate ganglion and facial nerve to the vestibulocochlear nerve in the bony facial canal. Patients with the Ramsay Hunt syndrome may also develop dysarthria or dysphagia indicative of lower cranial nerve involvement, reflecting the shared derivation of the facial, glossopharyngeal, and vagus nerves from the same branchial arch. MRI scanning, not usually performed in patients with the Ramsay Hunt syndrome, may reveal enhancement in the geniculate ganglion (Fig. 5-2) as well as in the intracanalicular and tympanic segments of the facial nerve during its course through the facial canal. These MRI changes may also be seen in patients with Bell's palsy. Although seemingly paradoxical, the Ramsay Hunt syndrome may occur in the absence of rash, as evidenced by the detection of VZV DNA in tears, saliva, or auricular skin scrapings in

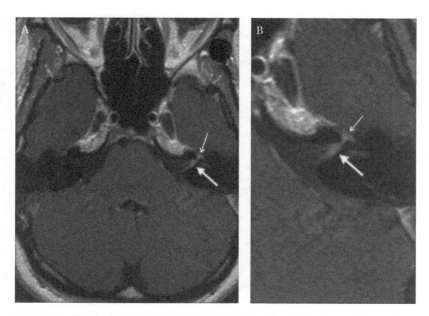

FIGURE 5-2 T1-weighted gadolinium-enhanced axial image showing the temporal bones at the level of the facial nerve in a patient with the Ramsay Hunt syndrome. Note enhancement in the geniculate ganglion (thin arrow) and of the facial nerve in the intracanalicular canal (thick arrow) and after enlargement of the photograph (B).

patients with peripheral facial palsy. While some controversy exists regarding the use of antivirals in patients with Bell's palsy, patients with Ramsay Hunt syndrome are best treated with valacyclovir, 1 gm, 3 times daily for 1 week. In addition, oral prednisone, 1 mg/kg of body weight, should be given for 5–7 days (no taper is necessary) to reduce facial nerve swelling in the small facial canal.

KEY POINTS TO REMEMBER

- Patients presenting with peripheral facial palsy should be examined for zoster lesions not only on the ipsilateral ear and tympanic membrane, but also on the palate and tongue.
- Treatment of the Ramsay Hunt syndrome should include antiviral agents and steroids.

Further Reading

Sweeney CJ, Gilden D. Ramsay Hunt syndrome. *J Neurol Neurosurg Psychiatry* 71:149–154, 2001.

Gilden D, Mahalingam R, Nagel MA, Pugazhenthi S, Cohrs RJ. The neurobiology of varicella zoster virus infection. *Neuropathol Appl Neurobiol 37*:441–463, 2011.

Gilden D. Functional anatomy of the facial nerve revealed by Ramsay Hunt syndrome. *Cleve Clin J Med 80*:78–79, 2013.

6 West Nile Virus Meningoencephalitis

A 41-year-old woman is hospitalized due to fever and confusion. One week earlier, she developed generalized headaches that gradually increased in intensity accompanied by mild photophobia and neck stiffness. Three days earlier, she thought she was mildly febrile. On the morning of admission, she awoke with shaking chills and a temperature of 104°F, and felt light-headed and fatigued. Her husband observes that she is confused. The patient resides in Connecticut. Three weeks earlier she had traveled to Missouri, where she walked in a wooded area and visited a zoo. A few days earlier she was visiting the New Jersey shore, where she was bitten by mosquitoes. She noticed ticks on her dog but not on herself. Multiple nonblanching, erythematous macular lesions are seen on both of her legs (Fig. 6-1). Neurological examination shows that she is alert and oriented, but easily confused and speaking in incomplete sentences. On her fourth hospital day, she develops asymmetric weakness of the arms and legs. The examination reveals lower motor neuron distribution weakness in all four extremities, worse in the right leg. Truncal weakness is also present, and she is unable to sit up in bed. DTRs are 1+ in the arms and absent in the legs. The CSF opening pressure is normal, and the CSF contains 210 WBCs (67 percent mononuclear, 33 percent neutrophils); the CSF protein is 110 mg percent and glucose is normal. MRI reveals bilateral deep-seated lesions in gray matter; the thalamus is most affected (Fig. 6-2).

What do you do now?

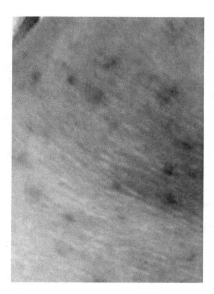

FIGURE 6-1 Skin lesions in West Nile virus infection. Multiple nonblanching, erythematous macular lesions are seen over the leg. (From Reznicek JE, Mason WJ, Kaul DR, Saint S, Bloch KC. Clinical problem-solving. Avoiding a rash diagnosis. *N Engl J Med 364*(5):466–471; 2011. Reprinted with permission from the Massachusetts Medical Society.)

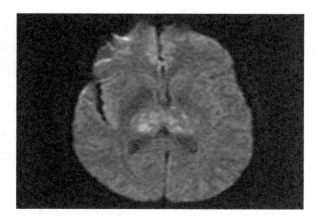

FIGURE 6-2 West Nile virus encephalitis. Diffusion-weighted MRI during the first week shows increased signal in the thalamus. (From Davis LE, DeBiasi R, Goade DE, Haaland KY, Harrington JA, Harnar JB, Pergam SA, King MK, DeMasters BK, Tyler KL. West Nile virus neuroinvasive disease. *Ann Neurol 60*(3):286–300; 2006. Reprinted with permission from John Wiley and Sons.)

The combined clinical, CSF, and MRI features are characteristic of meningoencephalitis. The skin rash and deep-seated lesions on MRI provide important clues to the causative agent. The skin rash could be produced by meningococcus, tick-borne rickettsial disease such as Rocky Mountain spotted fever, an enterovirus, Epstein Barr virus (EBV), or West Nile virus (WNV). Syphilis and Lyme disease also cause rash and meningoencephalitis. Deep-seated lesions on MRI are produced by EBV, WNV, togaviruses (e.g., Eastern equine encephalitis virus, St. Louis Encephalitis virus), but not by meningococcus, enteroviruses, or Rickettsia.

The CSF should be cultured for bacteria. Other important tests that should be performed on the CSF include a serological test for syphilis, anti-body testing for *Rickettsia rickettsii*, anti-IgM antibody and RT-PCR for WNV, PCR for enteroviruses, and PCR and antibody to EBV. While awaiting the results of diagnostic tests, the patient should receive broad-spectrum antimicrobial therapy to cover bacteria and rickettsial infection. Tests results revealed negative CSF culture and serology for syphilis, and no detectable antibody to *Rickettsia rickettsii* or EBV DNA or antibody in the CSF. PCR on CSF was negative for enterovirus and WNV, but the CSF was positive for anti-WNV IgM, thus clinching the diagnosis of WNV meningoencephalitis.

Virological confirmation of WNV infection is best provided by the detection in CSF or serum of anti-WNV IgM antibody. PCR for WNV is highly specific, but relatively insensitive compared with detection of anti-WNV IgM in CSF. WNV, an RNA virus of the genus *Flavivirus*, is transmitted by a mosquito vector from infected birds (e.g., crow, jays, grackles). WNV first appeared in the United States in 1999 and has emerged as the most common cause of epidemic meningoencephalitis in North America. Importantly, in addition to meningoencephalitis, WNV infection of the nervous system presents as acute flaccid asymmetric paralysis. Other presentations have included opsoclonus-myoclonus with cerebellar ataxia and unilateral brachial plexopathy. WNV must be considered as a cause of encephalomyelitis in organ transplant recipients. The CSF contains a pleocytosis with a median of more than 200 cells; often half of the cells are neutrophils. MRI may be normal, but when lesions are present, they are hyperintense on T2-weighting and have a predilection for deep gray matter structures, such as the thalamus, basal ganglia, brain stem, and cerebellum. There is no specific therapy of proven efficacy for treatment of WNV infection. Despite the efficacy of ribavirin, interferon-α, and WNV-specific antibodies against WNV in vitro, no clinical benefit was seen when these drugs were administered during WNV outbreaks.

KEY POINTS TO REMEMBER

- The neurological manifestations of WNV infection are protean and include meningoencephalitis or acute flaccid asymmetrical paralysis or combinations thereof.
- In addition to neurological disease, WNV infection produces a nonpruritic generalized maculopapular rash in ~20 percent of patients.
- Either mononuclear cells or neutrophils may predominate in CSF of patients with WNV infection of the nervous system.
- The single best test to confirm the diagnosis of WNV infection of the nervous system is detection of anti-WNV IgM in CSF.

Further Reading

Kleinschmidt-DeMasters BK, Marder BA, Levi ME, Laird SP, McNutt JT, Escott EJ, Everson GT, Tyler KL. Naturally acquired West Nile virus encephalomyelitis in transplant recipients: clinical, laboratory, diagnostic, and neuropathological features. *Arch Neurol 61*:1210-1220, 2004.

Davis LE, DeBiasi R, Goade DE, Haaland KY, Harrington JA, Harnar JB, Pergam SA, King MK, DeMasters BK, Tyler KL. West Nile virus neuroinvasive disease. *Ann Neurol 60*:286-300, 2006.

Tyler KL, Pape J, Goody RJ, Corkill M, Kleinschmidt-DeMasters BK. CSF findings in 250 patients with serologically confirmed West Nile virus meningitis and encephalitis. *Neurology 66*:361-365, 2006.

Progressive Outer Retinal Necrosis

A 38-year-old HIV-positive man complains of progressive, painless blurry vision in the left eye for the past 5 weeks. There are no other neurological or ocular symptoms. Six months ago, he developed left C4-distribution zoster. Two months ago, he experienced 3–4 transient episodes of right-sided weakness over a 1-week period. Brain MRI revealed bilateral cortical and subcortical lesions, a few of which enhanced. His visual acuity is 20/20 OD and 20/70 OS. Funduscopic examination reveals diffuse retinal hemorrhages and whitening with macular involvement (Fig. 7-1) in the left eye. The remainder of the neurologic examination is normal.

What do you do now?

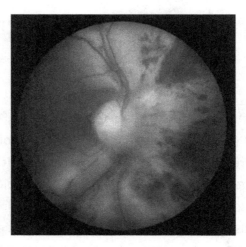

FIGURE 7-1 Progressive outer retinal necrosis. Note diffuse retinal hemorrhages and whitening with macular involvement. (From Nakamoto BK, Dorotheo EU, Biousse V, Tang RA, Schiffman JS, Newman NJ. Progressive outer retinal necrosis presenting with isolated optic neuropathy. *Neurology 63*(12):2423-2425; 2004. Reprinted with permission from Wolters Kluwer Health.)

The patient's visual loss and funduscopic changes are characteristic of progressive outer retinal necrosis (PORN). Most PORN is caused by varicella zoster virus (VZV), but herpes simplex virus (HSV) and cytomegalovirus (CMV) also produce identical retinitis. Each of these viruses is a DNA virus and a member of the human herpesvirus family.

PORN is more common in immunosuppressed individuals, particularly in AIDS patients with a CD4 count less than 10. PORN is often preceded or accompanied by zoster, aseptic meningitis, retrobulbar optic neuritis, central retinal artery occlusion, multifocal vasculopathy, or myelitis. Thus, the history of recent zoster with bilateral cortical and subcortical lesions in this patient, most likely due to VZV multifocal vasculopathy, strongly suggests VZV as the causative agent of the retinal necrosis. Nevertheless, because HIV+ individuals are susceptible to opportunistic infections by HSV or CMV, virological verification of the herpesvirus that caused PORN is required, since treatment for CMV-induced retinitis differs from that for VZV- or HSV-induced disease. PCR of aqueous fluid and of CSF for VZV, HSV, and CMV DNA should be performed immediately. In addition, the recent zoster and VZV vasculopathy in this patient warrants a brain MRI to assess the status of the cerebral lesions.

PORN usually presents with painless loss of vision, floaters, and constricted visual fields, with resultant retinal detachment. Multifocal, discrete opacified lesions begin in the outer retinal layers peripherally and/or posterior pole; only late in disease are inner retinal layers involved. PORN progresses rapidly, producing retinal gliosis with peripheral detachment, along with confluent retinal whitening and a broad band of satellite lesions (Fig. 7-2).

While awaiting the results of diagnostic tests, treatment should begin immediately. HSV and VZV are sensitive to acyclovir, whereas CMV infection requires treatment with ganciclovir and/or foscarnet (both more toxic). In this patient, I would begin with intravenous acyclovir for 2 weeks. Note that such treatment has given poor or inconsistent results, perhaps because such patients are often severely immunocompromised or may have PORN caused by CMV. Furthermore, even when acyclovir helps, VZV retinopathy

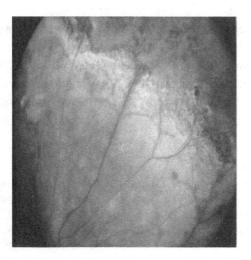

FIGURE 7-2 Herpetic retinitis in an HIV-infected person reveals three distinct zones of retinal infection: peripheral detachment of gliotic retina, confluent retinal whitening and a broad band of satellite lesions. (From Davis J. Acute retinal necrosis. In: Retinal Imaging (Huang D, Kaiser PK, Lowder CY, Traboulsi EI, eds). Philadelphia, PA: Mosby, Elsevier, Chap 43, 383-389, 2006. Reprinted with permission from Elsevier.)

may recur when drug is tapered or discontinued. If a rapid response is not seen with intravenous acyclovir, then ganciclovir and foscarnet (both given intravenously) should be considered. PORN patients treated with ganciclovir alone or in combination with foscarnet have a better final visual acuity than those treated with acyclovir or foscarnet. Intravitreal injection of ganciclovir and foscarnet, separately or together, has also been shown to reduce the risk of blindness. Finally, because HAART therapy in AIDS patients decreases the incidence of PORN, HAART therapy should be optimized in the patient.

Lack of a definitive regimen of antiviral agents for PORN is a challenge for the clinician. The neurologist must work closely with an ophthalmologist and infectious disease specialist to accurately diagnose the virological cause of PORN and to provide optimal treatment.

KEY POINTS TO REMEMBER

- Funduscopic features of PORN include retinal hemorrhages, areas of retinal whitening, and eventual retinal detachment.
- The most common cause of PORN is VZV, but HSV and CMV also produce PORN.
- No definitive regimen of antiviral agents to treat PORN has been determined. Patients with PORN should be managed by a team consisting of a neurologist, ophthalmologist, and infectious disease specialist.

Further Reading

Tran TH, Rozenberg F, Cassoux N, Rao NA, LeHoang P, Bodaghi B. Polymerase chain reaction analysis of aqueous humour samples in necrotizing retinitis. *Br J Ophthalomol* 87:79-83, 2003.

Davis J. Acute retinal necrosis. In: *Retinal Imaging* (Huang D, Kaiser PK, Lowder CY, Traboulsi El, eds). Philadelphia, PA: Mosby, Elsevier, Chap 43, 383-389, 2006.

8 Rabies

A 45-year-old man develops weakness and paresthesias in his left arm. A few days later, he is nearly paralyzed in all four extremities and can only wiggle his toes. During the next 2 days, his speech becomes thick and he has difficulty swallowing. There is no history of a recent cold, sore throat or diarrhea, tick bite, abdominal pain, trouble thinking, abnormal behavior, or double vision. Two months earlier he was vacationing in New Mexico and visited bat caves but does not recall being bitten by a bat. No ticks are found on his skin. Neurologic examination reveals a heightened sense of alertness with intact cognition. His tongue is weak bilaterally, and the jaw jerk and gag reflex are absent. The remaining cranial nerves are normal. There is a flaccid quadriplegia. All DTRs are absent. There is no sensory loss. The CSF opening pressure is normal, and there are 20 WBCs, all mononuclear. CSF protein is 60 mg percent. Both serum and CSF contain antirabies antibody.

What do you do now?

The patient presented with acute to subacute onset of quadriplegia and no sensory loss, followed by dysarthria and dysphagia. The most common cause of such a presentation is the Guillain-Barré syndrome. Acute paralysis can also be produced by toxins (n-hexane inhalation, thallium or arsenic poisoning), tick paralysis, porphyric neuropathy, diphtheria, and both West Nile virus and rabies virus. The absence of psychosis and abdominal pain reduces the likelihood of neuropathy from porphyria. There was no history of tick bite, and ticks were not found on his skin. The patient did not have an ophthalmoparesis usually seen in diphtheria and botulism. There was also no abdominal pain or skin rash to suggest arsenic poisoning, and no pain or hair loss as seen with thallium intoxication.

The history of exposure to bats in a cave mandates testing for antibody to rabies virus, which was positive. In conjunction with the clinical features, the diagnosis of "dumb" or paralytic rabies was established. The patient was treated with human rabies immune globulin and started on a 4-dose course of rabies vaccine, but died 10 days after receiving the second dose of vaccine. Autopsy revealed inflammation of the leptomeninges and perivascular mononuclear cell infiltrates in the cerebral parenchyma. Numerous infected neurons contained cytoplasmic eosinophilic inclusions (Negri bodies), a pathological hallmark of rabies (Fig. 8-1).

Rabies is an ancient disease cause by an RNA virus in the Rhabdovirus family. Wildlife accounts for most rabies in Asia and Africa, while bats are the main threat to humans in North America. Rabies virus is almost always transmitted by an animal bite, although aerosol transmission has been documented in laboratories or in caves containing millions of bats.

"Dumb" rabies accounts for 20 percent of all cases. The more common encephalitic ("furious") form is characterized by apathy, drowsiness, seizures, delirium, thrashing, headache, and a profuse flow of saliva due to spasmodic contraction of pharyngeal and laryngeal muscles precipitated by any attempt to eat or drink (hence, the term "hydrophobia"). Patients with the encephalitic form of rabies often have a high fever of 105°–107°F. The CSF in rabies usually contains a pleocytosis and increased protein.

The incubation period after a bite by a rabid animal varies from many days to a few months. The interval from a bite on the face until the onset of neurologic disease is shorter than after a bite on an extremity. Virtually all cases of rabies are fatal. Treatment is supportive. If someone has been bitten

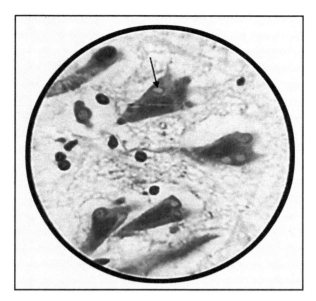

FIGURE 8-1 Rabies. Arrow points to one of many eosinophilic inclusions (Negri bodies) in the neuronal cytoplasm of a rabies virus-infected individual.

by a rabid animal, prophylaxis with rabies immune globulin and a course of vaccination should begin immediately.

KEY POINTS TO REMEMBER

- There are two forms of rabies. The encephalitic or "furious" form is characterized by apathy, drowsiness, seizures, delirium, thrashing, headache, and profuse saliva flow due to spasmodic contraction of pharyngeal and laryngeal muscles on attempts to eat or drink. The "dumb" form is characterized by rapidly progressive paralysis, dysarthria, and dysphagia that mimic the Guillain-Barré syndrome.
- All wildlife should be considered a potential source of rabies. If someone has been bitten by a rabid animal, prophylaxis with rabies immune globulin and a course of vaccination should begin immediately.

Further Reading

Jackson AC. Rabies. In: *Viral Infections of the Human Nervous System* (Jackson AC, ed). Basel: Springer, 87–114, 2012.

9 Cytomegalovirus Polyradiculoneuropathy

For 3 months a 45-year-old man with AIDS noted tingling sensations, often uncomfortable and more on the right side, extending from the gluteal area to the back of his thighs and calves. In the past 6 weeks his legs have weakened, and he has had difficulty walking and getting out of a chair. In the past 2 weeks he has had trouble emptying his bladder and had two episodes of fecal incontinence. Neurological examination reveals flaccid weakness in the lower extremities, worse on the right; thigh abduction and extension are most affected. There is asymmetric hypalgesia throughout the lower extremities with near-complete saddle-distribution anesthesia. The left patellar reflex is hypoactive, and the right patellar reflex and both Achilles reflexes are absent. Both plantar responses are flexor. Stool can be seen through his patulous anus, and there is no anal wink or bulbocavernosus reflex. A lumbosacral MRI reveals enhancement of some nerve roots, but no compressive or mass lesions. Two CSF exams are performed. The first CSF sample contains 210 WBCs, 90 percent mononuclear; CSF protein is 80 mg percent and glucose 40 mg percent. The second CSF contains 318 WBCs, 60 percent neutrophils; CSF protein is 105 mg percent and glucose 32 mg percent. Cytological examination of both CSFs reveals no malignant cells, and viral cultures and VDRL are negative. PCR analysis of CSF for the presence of cytomegalovirus (CMV), varicella zoster virus (VZV), and herpes simplex virus (HSV) DNA amplifies CMV DNA.

What do you do now?

The patient's symptoms and signs indicate involvement of nerve roots of the cauda equina. A lesion of the conus medullaris could also explain many of the clinical features, although conus lesions are usually characterized by early sphincter involvement and no leg weakness. The patient's sacral roots are the most severely affected, as evidenced by weak thigh abduction and extension, saddle anesthesia with loss of sphincter muscle control, and the absence of both an anal wink and bulbocavernosus reflex.

In AIDS patients, the leading causes of chronic polyradiculopathy are CMV, leptomeningeal lymphoma, and syphilis. VZV can also produce a polyradiculoneuropathy, even in the absence of rash, but the ganglioneuropathy would be painful, a feature not prominent in our patient. Two negative cytological examinations of the CSF for malignant cells makes leptomeningeal lymphoma unlikely, and a negative VDRL rules out subacute syphilitic involvement of the nerve roots. Positive PCR analysis of the CSF for CMV DNA clinched the diagnosis of CMV polyradiculoneuropathy.

CMV, a DNA virus, is one of eight human herpesviruses. After primary (first time) infection, virus becomes latent in lymphoid tissue. When acquired in utero, CMV can cause cytomegalic inclusion body disease in newborns with serious neurological complications that include microcephaly, deafness, and blindness. CMV is also one of the infectious agents associated with the Guillain-Barré syndrome (GBS). Another organism that is strongly associated with the axonal form of GBS is the bacterium *Campylobacter jejuni*. Importantly, antiganglioside antibodies in the axonal form of GBS cross-react with lipoligosaccharides in the outer membrane of *C. jejuni*, supporting the role of molecular mimicry in the pathogenesis of disease. Antiganglioside antibodies are also associated with GBS after CMV infection, but their relevance is still unknown.

Before the AIDS era, CMV infection of the adult nervous system was rare. Now, however, AIDS patients develop infection of ependymal cells lining the ventricular system, with gait disturbances, mental status changes, and hydrocephalus. Nonetheless, the most common neurological problem caused by CMV in AIDS patients is polyradiculoneuropathy.

Note that in CMV polyradiculoneuropathy, either mononuclear cells or neutrophils may predominate in the CSF, the latter perhaps reflecting chronic active disease. Hypoglycorrachia is also common in patients with CMV polyradiculoneuropathy. On one occasion, when no measurable glucose was detected in the CSF, the hospital technician called to be sure that CSF, not water, had been sent to the clinical laboratory! CMV infection requires treatment with foscarnet and ganciclovir, but the prognosis is poor. Furthermore, polyradiculoneuropathy often recurs when antiviral therapy is discontinued. Pathological changes reveal necrosis with inflammatory infiltrates and focal vascililtis of nerve roots.

KEY POINTS TO REMBEMBER

- In AIDS patients, the leading causes of a polyradiculopathy are CMV, leptomeningeal lymphoma, and syphilis.
- A positive CSF PCR for CMV DNA verifies the diagnosis of CMV polyradiculoneuropathy.
- CMV polyradiculoneuropathy is usually chronic, and either mononuclear cells or neutrophils may predominate in the CSF.
- Hypoglycorrachia is common in patients with CMV polyradiculoneuropathy.

Further Reading

Eidelberg D, Sotrel A, Vogel H, Walker P, Kleefield J, Crumpacker CS 3rd. Progressive polyradiculopathy in acquired immune deficiency syndrome. *Neurology 36*:912-916, 1986.

Achim CL, Nagra RM, Wang, R, Nelson JA, Wiley CA. Detection of cytomegalovirus in cerebrospinal fluid autopsy specimens from AIDS patients. *J Infect Dis 169*:623-662, 1994.

10 Varicella Zoster Virus Myelopathy

A 56-year-old woman develops left ophthalmic-distribution zoster. Despite treatment with famciclovir 500 mg 3 times daily for 1 week, facial pain persists for a year (postherpetic neuralgia). Two months after the onset of zoster, she develops a Lhermitte's symptom and left leg weakness. After another 2 months, she notes urinary urgency, rectal paresthesias, and loss of sensation during stool evacuation and when wiping herself. Neurological examination reveals a spastic paraparesis, worse on the left, hyperactive DTRs, bilateral leg clonus, and a left extensor plantar response; all sensory modalities are intact. Cervical MRI reveals an enhancing lesion in the midcervical spinal cord (Fig. 10-1, left). CSF is acellular and CSF protein is normal. The following studies are negative or normal: ESR, CRP, serologic test for syphilis, serum vitamin B12, angiotensin-converting enzyme levels, ANA, HIV and Lyme antibodies, NMO-IgG, anti-SSA or -SSB antibodies, and visual evoked responses.

Six months later, she develops increasing leg weakness and urinary incontinence. Neurological examination reveals a spastic paraparesis with bilateral extensor plantar responses. Cervical MRI reveals new lesions in the upper cervical spinal cord and at the cervicomedullary lesion (Fig. 10-1, right). A repeat CSF examination is normal. The CSF is negative for PCR-amplifiable herpes simplex virus (HSV)-1, HSV-2, and varicella zoster virus (VZV) DNA, but positive for anti-VZV IgG antibody, and the serum/CSF ratio of anti-VZV IgG is reduced compared to ratios for total IgG and albumin, consistent with intrathecal synthesis of anti-VZV IgG antibody.

What do you do now?

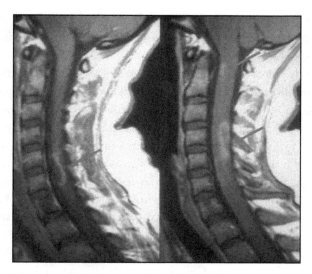

FIGURE 10-1 VZV myelopathy. Cervical MRI. Arrows point to enhancing lesions in the midcervical spinal cord (left), and 6 months later, in the upper cervical spinal cord and cervicomedullary junction (right). (From Gilden DH, Beinlich BR, Rubinstien EM, Stommel E, Swenson R, Rubinstien D, Mahalingam R. Varicella-zoster virus myelitis: an expanding spectrum. *Neurology* 44(10):1818-1823; 1994. Reprinted with permission from Wolters Kluwer Health.)

The patient has VZV myelitis and should be treated immediately with intravenous acyclovir, 10–15 mg/kg for 14 days. Note that the test confirming diagnosis is the presence of anti-VZV IgG antibody in CSF. The superiority of detection of anti-VZV antibody in the absence of amplifiable VZV DNA in CSF to diagnose VZV-produced neurological disease has also been demonstrated in VZV vasculopathy. Other salient features of VZV myelopathy include its chronic, protracted, and even recurrent nature (as in the case herein). Like other VZV-produced neurological disorders such as vasculopathy, cerebellitis, meningoencephalitis, polyneuritis cranialis, retinitis, and radiculopathy (classic zoster sine herpete), VZV myelopathy may also precede zoster rash and develop in the absence of rash.

VZV myelopathy manifests in various ways. One form is a self-limiting, monophasic disorder, characterized by acute spastic paraparesis, with or without sensory features and sphincter problems. This so-called postinfectious myelitis usually occurs in immunocompetent individuals days to weeks after acute varicella or zoster. Its pathogenesis is unknown. The CSF usually contains a mild mononuclear pleocytosis, with normal or slightly elevated protein. Steroids are used to treat these patients, although some improve spontaneously.

Currently, most VZV myelopathy presents as zoster-associated progressive myelitis. In immunocompromised individuals and especially in HIV-positive individuals, disease can be fatal. MRI reveals longitudinal serpiginous enhancing lesions. Pathological and virological analyses of the spinal cord from fatal cases have shown frank invasion of VZV in the parenchyma, and in some instances, spread of virus to adjacent nerve roots. Not surprisingly, some patients respond favorably to antiviral therapy. Early diagnosis and aggressive treatment with intravenous acyclovir have been helpful, even in immunocompromised patients. The benefit of steroids in addition to antiviral agents is unknown. In the absence of rash, the diagnosis of VZV myelopathy is confirmed by the presence of VZV DNA in CSF, anti-VZV IgM in serum or CSF, or anti-VZV IgG in CSF in patients with progressive or recurrent myelopathy.

Finally, VZV can also produce spinal cord infarction, identified by diffusion-weighted MRI and confirmed virologically, and thus can cause stroke in the spinal cord as well as in the brain.

KEY POINTS TO REMEMBER

- VZV myelopathy is often chronic, protracted, and recurrent.
- Myelopathy caused by VZV may precede zoster rash or develop with no history of zoster rash.
- To diagnose VZV vasculopathy in the absence of rash, serum should be examined for anti-VZV IgM antibody and CSF should be examined for PCR-amplifiable VZV DNA and anti-VZV IgG or anti-VZV IgM antibody. In patients with clinical features of myelopathy, the presence of anti-VZV IgM antibody in serum or detection of VZV DNA, anti-VZV IgM, or IgG in CSF confirms the diagnosis of VZV myelopathy.

Further Reading

Gilden DH, Beinlich BR, Rubinstien EM, Stommel E, Swenson R, Rubinstein D, Mahalingam R. Varicella zoster virus myelitis: an expanding spectrum. *Neurology* 44:1818-1823, 1994.

de Silva SM, Mark AS, Gilden DH, Mahalingam R, Balish M, Sandbrink F, Houff S. Zoster myelitis: improvement with antiviral therapy in two cases *Neurology 47*: 929–931, 1996.

Morita Y, Osaki Y, Doi Y, Forghani B, Gilden DH. Chronic active VZV infection manifesting as zoster sine herpete, zoster paresis and myelopathy. *J Neurol Sci 212*: 7–9, 2003.

Orme HT, Smith G, Nagel MA, Bert RJ, Mickelson TS, Gilden DH. VZV spinal cord infarction identified by diffusion-weighted MRI (DWI). *Neurology 69*:398–400, 2007.

Gilden D, Nagel MA, Ransohoff RM, Cohrs RJ, Mahalingam R, Tanabe JL. Recurrent varicella zoster virus myelopathy. *J Neurol Sci 276* :196–198, 2009.

Subacute Sclerosing Panencephalitis

The parents of an 8-year-old boy whose growth and development have been normal are contacted by his 3rd grade teacher who says that "he is failing in school work." A few months later, he starts falling to the left, begins to use only his left hand and responds to questions with only "Yes" or "No." Within another 2 months, he becomes aphasic and incontinent and develops a right hemiparesis. In the next 6 months, he becomes quadriplegic and experiences generalized convulsions. On examination, he is unresponsive to verbal stimuli and withdraws his limbs only in response to deep pain. All four extremities are rigid. DTRs are hyperactive and both plantar responses are extensor. An MRI scan reveals diffuse symmetric involvement of the periventricular and subcortical white matter in the frontal and parietal regions bilaterally (Fig. 11-1). An EEG is markedly abnormal, with a diffuse generalized delta rhythm of high amplitude. The CSF contains 15 WBCs, all mononuclear, with a normal CSF protein and glucose. IgG synthesis is markedly increased and there are 18 oligoclonal bands. Serum and CSF antibody to HIV is negative.

What do you do now?

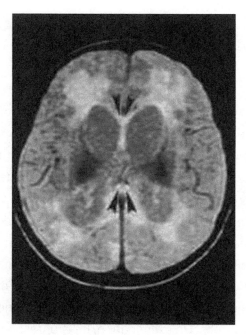

FIGURE 11-1 Subacute sclerosing panencephalitis. T2-weighted axial image demonstrates diffuse symmetrical involvement of the periventricular and subcortical white matter in the frontal and parietal regions bilaterally. Arrowheads indicate diffuse involvement of the corpus callosum. (From Anlar B, Saatçi I, Köse G, Yalaz K. MRI findings in subacute sclerosing panencephalitis. *Neurology 47*(5):1278-1283; 1996. Reprinted with permission from Wolters Kluwer Health.)

The clinical diagnosis as evidenced by progressive deterioration in mental status and increasing motor deficit with a CSF pleocytosis is chronic encephalitis. Because granulomatous disease is often chronic, disorders such as Lyme disease, tuberculous meningitis, and fungal meningitis must be ruled out. The patient is too young to have acquired syphilis. The absence of headache, fever, neutrophils, and decreased glucose in the CSF argue against tuberculous or fungal meningitis. Also, the patient is not immunocompromised and did not have any RBCs in the CSF, further reducing the likelihood of fungal meningitis. A paraneoplastic encephalitis would not be expected to last so long without evidence of cancer, such as in a child with neuroblastoma, although there is one report of a 20-month interval between the onset of neurological symptoms and tumor detection.

The critical laboratory test required in this patient is a search for antibody to measles virus in serum and CSF. Conventional testing is for either complement-fixation or hemagglutination-inhibition antibody (HAI) against measles virus. In this patient, the HAI titer was 1:1096 in serum and 1:128 in CSF, confirming the diagnosis of subacute sclerosing panencephalitis (SSPE) and obviating brain biopsy.

SSPE occurs primarily in children and teenagers, with most cases in young boys. In about half of patients, measles occurs before the age of 2 years and SSPE develops about 7 years later. The first signs are usually mental and behavioral changes. The patient becomes apathetic, irritable, and sometimes psychotic. School work deteriorates due to poor memory and general intellectual decline. Focal neurologic signs then ensue, such as dysphasia, hemiparesis, and involuntary movements, both athetoid and choreiform. Visual abnormalities are common and are bilateral and homonymous when a visual pathway or the striate cortex is involved or monocular when the macula is involved. Major, minor, myoclonic, and partial complex seizures all may occur in SSPE, with myoclonic seizures being the most frequent. Myoclonus frequently heralds the late stages of disease as the patient becomes increasingly demented and stuporous and as decorticate rigidity develops. There is no pain, headache, or fever. Increased and often rising levels of anti–measles virus antibody are found in serum and CSF. A modest pleocytosis of 5–20 mononuclear cells is often present. The percentage of CSF IgG in total protein is increased; values as high 40–50 percent are common (normal 3–13 percent). In addition, oligoclonal bands are seen. Most CSF oligoclonal IgG is directed against measles virus. The EEG may help in diagnosis. Periodic bisynchronous, symmetric 2- to 4-Hz high-amplitude delta-waves may occur every 5–7 seconds. Periodic transients are also seen in diffuse CNS disorders, such as the cerebral lipidoses or anoxia, conditions that are readily distinguishable from SSPE. MRI brain scanning reveals extensive demyelination with cortical atrophy late in disease. More fulminant cases ("acute" SSPE) have been described in patients who have macular disease before the onset of CNS involvement. Disease is always fatal. No antiviral agent has proven to be effective.

Pathologic findings in SSPE include diffuse encephalitis of both gray and white matter (panencephalitis) including the brain stem, with perivascular cuffing of mononuclear cells and proliferation of both macroglia and microglia. Cowdry type A intranuclear inclusion bodies are seen in neurons, astrocytes, and oligodendroctyes. Ultrastructural examination reveals the presence of paramyxovirus nucleocapsids.

SSPE results from defective measles virus. There is no evidence of an altered host immune response to virus. Since the era of widespread measles vaccine use, the incidence of SSPE has declined from 5–10 cases per million to about 0.5–1 case per million.

The only other viruses that cause chronic progressive encephalitis are rubella virus and HIV. Progressive rubella panencephalitis is a rare CNS disorder that develops about a decade after congenital rubella infection. Fewer than 10 cases have been described. The clinical features are similar to those of SSPE (progressive mental and motor deterioration, ataxia, chorea, and myoclonic seizures). The CSF reveals a mild mononuclear pleocytosis with increased protein and IgG levels. High titers of antibody to rubella virus are in serum and CSF, distinguishing this disorder from SSPE. Another chapter in this book is devoted to the clinical, CSF, and imaging features of HIV encephalitis.

KEY POINTS TO REMEMBER

- Chronic progressive encephalitis is most often seen in tuberculous and fungal infections, Lyme disease, and syphilis. The only viruses that cause chronic progressive encephalitis are HIV, measles, and rubella virus.
- Oligoclonal bands are found in chronic progressive encephalitis caused by measles virus, rubella virus, and HIV.

Further Reading

Gilden DH, Rorke LB, Tanaka R. Acute SSPE. *Arch Neurol 32*:644-646, 1975.

Gilden DH. Slow virus diseases of the CNS. *Postgrad Med 73*:99-118, 1983.

Anlar B, Saatçi I, Köse G, Yalaz K. MRI findings in subacute sclerosing panencephalitis. *Neurology 47*:1278-1283, 1996.

12   Eastern Equine Encephalitis

In the middle of the summer in New England, a 49-year-old woman is hospitalized for fever and confusion. One week earlier, she told her family she felt sick. In the next few days, she became extremely fatigued and lethargic and developed headache and aching in her legs. The day before hospitalization, she appeared to be listless, and her husband noticed that her skin was hot. Later that day, she became confused. On examination, she is lethargic and disoriented with slow and inappropriate responses to questions. Her temperature is 102°F, her pulse is 110/minute and respirations are 28 breaths/minute. Her neck is supple. Cranial nerves are normal. Tone in the arms and legs is normal, and she moves all her extremities spontaneously. DTRs are brisk, and there are no pathologic reflexes. A few hours after arrival to the hospital, she has a tonic-clonic seizure that lasts for 30 seconds. After the seizure, she becomes increasingly somnolent and does not respond to painful stimuli. She is intubated immediately. CBC reveals a hemoglobin of 12.3, WBC count of 17,500, 90 percent neutrophils, and platelets are normal. All lab chemistries are normal. A brain MRI scan shows increased signal in subcortical white matter, the thalami, and substantia nigra (Fig. 12-1). The CSF is clear, and CSF opening pressure is normal. The CSF contains 1,423 WBCs,

60 percent neutrophils, 40 percent mononuclear; CSF protein is 150 mg percent, and glucose 82 mg percent. Gram stain on CSF reveals abundant neutrophils but no bacteria, and CSF culture is negative. PCR for herpes simplex virus (HSV) and varicella zoster virus (VZV) DNA, and enterovirus RNA is negative. Lyme and West Nile virus (WNV) antibody in both serum and CSF are negative.

The woman lives in a rural wooded area of Connecticut. She has not traveled internationally in the past decade. She has no allergies or unusual exposures to chemicals or toxic materials. She has no pets and there is no known direct exposure to ticks, rodents, wild game, or birds. She drinks alcohol socially, but does not smoke or use illicit drugs. She swims in a chlorinated outdoor pool and has been bitten by mosquitoes.

What do you do now?

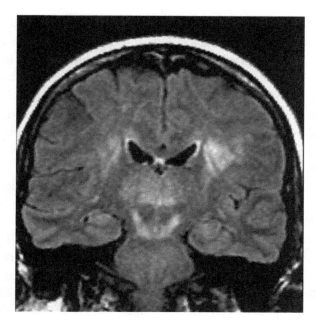

FIGURE 12-1 Eastern equine encephalitis. MRI scan shows increased signal in subcortical white matter, thalami, and substantia nigra.

While summer in New England offers beaches, boating, and swimming, it can also lead to arthropod-borne virus (arbovirus) diseases. The patient had a febrile illness with headache, mental status changes, and lethargy that progressed to coma. The acute onset of disease, particularly with neutrophils in the CSF, is a feature of acute bacterial meningitis, which must always be ruled out when fever is complicated by headache, stiff neck, and rapidly progressing neurologic disease. Thus, it is essential to begin broad-spectrum antibiotics immediately to counter the major potential bacterial pathogens, such as *Haemophilus influenzae*, *Neisseria meningitidis*, *Streptococcus pneumoniae*, and *Listeria monocytogenes*. However the normal gram stain and absence of bacterial growth in CSF made infection with one of these organisms unlikely. Lyme disease must also be considered in this setting, since infection with *Borrelia burgdorferi* is common in New England during the summer and a tick bite might well have gone unrecognized by the patient. Neurologic features are often the first manifestations of Lyme disease and the patient may not have other findings of erythema migrans or arthritis; however, fulminant encephalitis is not characteristic of Lyme disease. The imaging changes are not characteristic of HSV-1, HSV-2, or VZV encephalitis, and negative PCRs confirmed the absence of those viruses. West Nile virus (WNV) infection must be considered, especially in the summer and particularly with deep-seated lesions on MRI, but was likely ruled out in this patient since a search for antibodies against WNV in serum and CSF as well as PCR for WNV RNA were negative. Lyme disease was also ruled out by the absence of antibody directed against *B. burgdorferi* in serum and CSF. Finally, PCR for enterovirus RNA was negative.

The history of mosquito bites further suggests an arbovirus infection. Arboviruses are members of the Togavirus family, among which are the viruses that cause Eastern equine encephalitis (EEE), Western equine encephalitis (WEE), Venezuelan equine encephalitis (VEE), St. Louis encephalitis, and other encephalitides. Many cases of arbovirus encephalitis are seen in children. EEE is the most neuropathogenic arbovirus transmitted in the United States. Most cases in humans generally occur in the Northeast between July and October. Incubation periods generally exceed a week and are followed by a prodrome of fever, headache, and other influenza-like symptoms as seen in this patient. Once neurologic manifestations develop, deterioration is rapid; seizures and focal neurologic signs including cranial nerve palsies are common, as are peripheral blood leukocytosis and often hyponatremia. Neutrophils may predominate in the CSF pleocytosis, and elevated protein levels are characteristic, whereas glucose is normal. MRI characteristically shows increased signal intensity in deep-seated structures, such as the basal ganglia and thalamus, and mass effects are also common. Diagnosis is confirmed by detection of IgM antibodies against EEE virus or of virus-specific RNA in CSF. In this patient, both the serum and CSF were found to contain IgM antibodies against EEE virus. The patient did not die but was left severely impaired, with cognitive changes and spasticity. There are no approved antiviral agents for EEE virus or any other arboviruses.

- Arbovirus encephalitides (EEE, WEE, VEE, etc.) are common in summer and early fall.
- The MRI in arbovirus encephalitis most often reveals changes in deep-seated structures such as the basal ganglia, thalamus, and cerebellum.
- A CSF pleocytosis in arbovirus encephalitis often reveals a predominance of neutrophils.

Further Reading

Deresiewicz RL, Thaler SJ, Hsu L, Zamani AA. Clinical and neuroradiographic manifestations of eastern equine encephalitis. *NEJM 336*:1867–1874, 1997.

13 Human Herpesvirus-6 Encephalitis

Three weeks after stem cell transplantation for acute myeloblastic leukemia, a 20-year-old man develops short-term memory loss and insomnia. Neurologic examination reveals an alert patient who can answer questions regarding remote events, but cannot remember daily events and performs poorly on memory testing. Over the next few weeks, he becomes increasingly confused and agitated. He has one major motor seizure that is successfully treated with anticonvulsants. Blood glucose, liver and renal function studies, and a urine toxicology screen are normal. CSF is clear and acellular; CSF protein is 110 mg percent, and glucose is normal. MRI reveals an increased T2 signal and mild swelling of the left hippocampus (Fig. 13-1). CSF is sent for PCR evidence of herpes simplex virus (HSV)-1 and -2, varicella zoster virus (VZV), Epstein-Barr virus (EBV) and human herpesvirus-6 (HHV-6) DNA.

What do you do now?

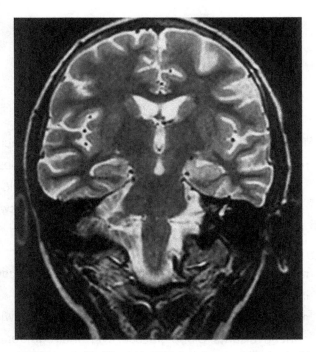

FIGURE 13-1 HHV-6 encephalitis. T2-weighted MRI shows increased signal and mild swelling of the left hippocampus. (From Wainwright MS, Martin PL, Morse RP, Lacaze M, Provenzale JM, Coleman RE, Morgan MA, Hulette C, Kurtzberg J, Bushnell C, Epstein L, Lewis DV. Human herpesvirus 6 limbic encephalitis after stem cell transplantation. *Ann Neurol 50*(5):612–619; 2001. Reprinted with permission from John Wiley and Sons.)

This immunosuppressed patient developed a subacute progressive encephalopathy. The CSF was acellular, and the MRI revealed increased signal in the hippocampus. Multiple disorders can produce a subacute encephalopathy. A toxic or metabolic disorder was ruled out by normal lab chemistries and a normal toxicology screen. The MRI abnormality was not consistent with cerebral hemorrhage. The increased signal in the hippocampus could indicate an early tumor or limbic encephalitis due to virus or a paraneoplastic syndrome. The latter is unlikely in a transplant recipient. Instead, the increased signal and edema is most consistent with inflammation due to infection by a herpesvirus such as HSV-1 or -2, VZV, or HHV-6. HSV-1 or -2 infections in the temporal lobe usually produce acute hemorrhagic necrosis with massive edema that evolves over a few days, and disease does not usually progress for weeks. PCR was positive for amplifiable HHV-6 DNA in CSF. Despite treatment with a multitude of antiviral agents, the patient continued to deteriorate and died. Autopsy revealed multiple microglial nodules throughout the brain, and immunohistochemistry revealed the presence of HHV-6 viral antigen.

HHV-6, a DNA virus and one of eight human herpesviruses, was first isolated from patients with lymphoproliferative disorders in 1986. HHV-6 isolates are classified as variants A (HHV-6A) and B (HHV-6B). HHV-6B is the major cause of exanthema subitum, while no disease has yet been associated with HHV-6A. Exanthema subitum (roseola infantum or "sixth disease") is characterized by sudden high fever that lasts for a few days, usually in infants. With defervescence, a macular rash appears over the trunk and face, ultimately spreading to the legs. Seizures are commonly associated with HHV-6 infections. HHV-6 can reactivate from latency in T cells after bone marrow or solid organ transplantation and in AIDS patients. HHV-6 also causes encephalitis in immunocompetent individuals. Unlike CNS infection caused by other herpesviruses, a CSF pleocytosis is often not seen in HHV-6 encephalitis, particularly in immunocompromised individuals. There are several reports of successful treatment of HHV-6 encephalitis with foscarnet and ganciclovir, but no clinical trial data are available.

KEY POINTS TO REMEMBER

- HHV-6 encephalitis occurs in both children and adults and is often fatal, particularly in immunocompromised individuals.
- In HHV-6 encephalitis, seizures, memory loss, insomnia, and agitation are more common than focal motor deficit.
- In HHV-6 encephalitis, the CSF is often acellular.
- In HHV-6 encephalitis, the MRI is either normal, or may show increased signal and mild swelling of the medial temporal lobe.

Further Reading

Salahuddin SA, Ablashi DV, Markham PD, Josephs SF, Sturzenegger S, Kaplan M, Halligan G, Biberfeld P, Wong-Staal F, Kramarsky B, Gallo RC. Isolation of a new virus, HBLV, in patients with lymphoproliferative disorders. *Science* 234:596-600, 1986.

Yamanishi K, Okuno T, Shiraki K, Takahashi M, Kondo T, Asano Y, Kurata T. Identification of human herpesvirus-6 as a causal agent for exanthema subitum. *Lancet* *8594*:1065–1067, 1988.

Wainwright MS, Martin PL, Morse RP, Lacaze M, Provenzale JM, Coleman RE, Morgan MA, Hulette C, Kurtzberg J, Bushnell C, Epstein L, Lewis DV. Human herpesvirus 6 limbic encephalitis after stem cell transplantation. *Ann Neurol 50*:612–619, 2001.

Tyler KL, Gilden D. Clinical management of viral encephalitis. In: *Neurotropic Viral Infections* (Reiss CS, ed). Cambridge, UK: Cambridge University Press, Chap 9, 347-361, 2008.

14   Zoster Sine Herpete

For more than 1 year a 64-year-old man has been
experiencing severe left-sided thoracic radicular pain
that extends from his back to the anterior surface of
his chest over the nipple area. Pain is relentless, sharp,
and lancinating. Pain is not affected by position, time
of day, or Valsalva maneuvers. A light touch over the
area elicits pain (allodynia). He has always been in good
general health. There is no history of diabetes. No rash,
hyperpigmentation, or depigmentation is seen over the
affected area. The neurological examination is normal
except for T4-distribution allodynia. A thoracic spine
MRI is normal. The CSF is acellular and the CSF protein
is normal. PCR of the CSF reveals amplifiable varicella
zoster virus (VZV), but not herpes simplex virus DNA.

What do you do now?

Prolonged localized radicular pain occurs in diabetes and is also produced by irritation or compression of a nerve root by a disk (unusual in the thoracic region) or by an epidural tumor (e.g., lymphoma, neurofibroma, or extradural meningioma). The patient is not diabetic. The normal MRI rules out an extradural lesion. The absence of a CSF pleocytosis and the normal CSF protein helps to rule out a chronic inflammatory or neoplastic disorder. The combination of T4 dermatomal-distribution radicular pain, absence of any structural lesion irritating the left T4 nerve root, and presence of VZV DNA in CSF clinches the diagnosis of zoster sine herpete.

Historically, the notion of zoster sine herpete was supported by multiple case descriptions of patients with zoster who also experienced radicular pain without rash in a different dermatome. Today, most neurologists view zoster sine herpete as radicular pain without rash in a person with no history of zoster. Virological confirmation for the nosological entity of zoster sine herpete was provided by amplification of VZV DNA from the CSF of two men over age 60, each of whom had thoracic-distribution radicular pain for 1–2 years in the absence of rash followed by a gratifying response in both patients after treatment with intravenous acyclovir, 10–15 mg/kg for 2 weeks. Later cases of zoster sine herpete were virologically confirmed by detection of VZV DNA in blood mononuclear cells and anti-VZV IgG in CSF. A more recent case involved a patient who developed radicular pain without rash in the same dermatome as zoster 1 year earlier; zoster sine herpete was confirmed by the detection of anti-VZV IgG antibody in CSF and a favorable response to antiviral therapy.

Overall, the CSF of patients who develop intractable radicular pain and show no evidence of compressive root disease should be examined for both VZV DNA and anti-VZV IgG antibody. The presence of either confirms the diagnosis of zoster sine herpete. While zoster sine herpete may respond to oral valacyclovir, patients may need treatment with intravenous acyclovir, 10–15 mg per kg, 3 times daily for 2 weeks. Virus reactivation with or without rash is due primarily to loss of cell-mediated immunity to VZV. In fact, the significantly lower cell-mediated immunity to VZV in diabetics compared with age-stratified healthy individuals in a large population-based study suggests that diabetes mellitus is a risk factor for herpes zoster, further complicating the differential diagnosis of prolonged radicular pain in patients with diabetes. Because radiculopathy without rash in some diabetics may be caused by VZV, these patients should be evaluated for both VZV DNA and anti-VZV IgG antibody in CSF and may need prolonged treatment with antiviral agents.

KEY POINTS TO REMEMBER

- Confirmation of zoster sine herpete (radicular pain without rash) requires detection of VZV DNA in CSF or in blood mononuclear cells or anti-VZV IgG antibody in CSF.
- Because cell-mediated immune responses to VZV are more impaired in diabetics than in normal individuals, the CSF should be examined for VZV DNA and anti-VZV IgG antibody before relegating chronic radicular pain without rash to diabetic radiculopathy.
- Patients with zoster sine herpete will likely require intravenous treatment with acyclovir.

Further Reading

Lewis GW. Zoster sine herpete. *Br Med J 2*:418–421, 1958.

Gilden DH, Wright RR, Schneck SA, Gwaltney JM Jr, Mahalingam R. Zoster sine herpete a clinical variant. *Ann Neurol 35*:530–533, 1994.

Amlie-Lefond C, Mackin GA, Ferguson M, Wright RR, Mahalingam R, Gilden DH. Another case of virologically confirmed zoster sine herpete, with electrophysiologic correlation. *J NeuroVirol 2*:136–138, 1996.

Okamoto S, Hata A, Sadaoka K, Yamanishi K, Mori Y. Comparison of varicella zoster virus-specific immunity of patients with diabetes mellitus and healthy individuals. *J Infect Dis 200*:1606–1610, 2009.

Blumenthal DT, Shacham-Shmueli E, Bokstein F, Schmid DS, Cohrs RJ, Nagel MA, Mahalingam R, Gilden D. Zoster sine herpete virological verification by detection of anti-VZV IgG antibody in CSF. *Neurology 76*:484–485, 2011.

Wolf J, Nagel MA, Mahalingam R, Cohrs RJ, Schmid SD, Gilden D. Chronic active varicella zoster virus infection. *Neurology 79*:828–829, 2012.

15 Human T-lymphotropic Virus-1 (HTLV-1) Myelopathy

A 51-year-old man noticed gait difficulty. Within 3 years, his legs were weak and stiff, and he became incontinent of urine and feces. Two years later, he could not walk without a cane, and after 2 more years, he was wheelchair-bound. He never developed pain or paresthesias. There was no history of homosexuality, intravenous drug abuse, or blood transfusion. He was born in Jamaica and moved to the United States at age 35. The neurologic examination reveals a normal mental status. Cranial nerves and upper extremity strength are normal, although tone is mildly increased in the arms. His legs are spastic with spontaneous clonus and weakness of all muscle groups. DTRs are hyperactive in the arms and legs, and both plantar responses are extensor. Abdominal reflexes are absent. All sensory modalities are intact.

CSF is clear and contains 15 WBCs, all mononuclear; CSF protein is 24 mg percent. CSF IgG constitutes 17 percent of total protein (normal 3–13 percent), and there are 7 oligoclonal bands. MRI scan of the spinal cord reveals several irregular linear focal areas of enhancement along the posterior aspect of the thoracic spinal cord (Fig. 15-1). Serum vitamin B12 and folic acid levels are normal. A serologic test for syphilis is negative. Serum and CSF angiotensin-converting enzyme levels are normal. No antibody to HIV or varicella zoster virus (VZV) is detected in serum of CSF, and PCR for VZV DNA in CSF is negative. High antibody titers to human T-lymphotropic virus 1 (HTLV-1) are found in both serum and CSF.

What do you do now?

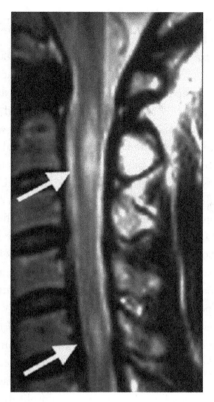

FIGURE 15-1 HTLV-1 myelopathy. T2-weighted MRI shows high intensity signal (arrows) in the cervical spinal cord. (From Umehara F, Tokunaga N, Hokezu Y, Hokonohara E, Yoshishige K, Shiraishi T, Okubo R, Osame M. Relapsing cervical cord lesions on MRI in patients with HTLV-I-associated myelopathy. *Neurology66*(2):289; 2006. Reprinted with permission from Wolters Kluwer Health.)

The patient has a chronic progressive inflammatory myelopathy with high titers of HTLV-1 antibody in serum and CSF, confirming the diagnosis of HTLV-1 myelopathy. Unlike HIV, the most common retrovirus that causes neurologic disease, the HTLV-1 retrovirus causes disease in only about 5 percent of infected people. HTLV-1 is estimated to infect 10 million people worldwide. Endemic areas of HTLV-1 myelopathy include Japan, central and west Africa, the Caribbean, Central and South America, and the Middle East. In Europe and North America, the virus is found primarily in immigrants from endemic areas, as seen in the patient herein, who was born and raised in Jamaica, as well as in some communities of intravenous drug abusers.

HTLV-1 myelopathy, also known as HAM (HTLV-1-associated myelopathy) and TSP (tropical spastic paraparesis), is characterized by slowly progressive spastic paraparesis with gait and sphincter disturbances. High antibody titers to HTLV-1 are seen in both serum and CSF. The CSF is either acellular or may contain a lymphocytic pleocytosis with increased IgG and oligoclonal bands. MRI often reveals increased signal in the spinal cord and less often in brain white matter. Although retroviral particles are not seen in infected tissue, HTLV-I proviral DNA and HTLV-1 proteins have been detected in affected spinal cord. Blood transfusions, contaminated needles, and sexual contact are sources of infectious virus. There is no definitive treatment for HTLV-1 myelopathy, although a double-blind multicenter study on the effect of treatment with natural interferon-α indicated a significant therapeutic benefit. Treatment with the nucleotide analog lamivudine reduces the virus load, but the clinical impact of such treatment is unknown.

Importantly, a person infected with HTLV-1 will have about a 5 percent lifetime risk of developing adult T-cell leukemia (ATL). More than half of ATL patients will have neurologic complications during the course of disease that include an altered state of consciousness due to hypercalcemia, dementia, seizures, focal deficits with long tract signs, cranial nerve deficits, meningitis, and neuropathy. Many of these complications are associated with tumor cell invasion.

KEY POINTS TO REMEMBER

- HTLV-1 is a cause of chronic progressive myelopathy.
- Virological confirmation comes from detection of high titers of HTLV-1 antibody in serum and CSF of patients.
- In HTLV-1 myelopathy, the CSF may be acellular or exhibit a modest pleocytosis.
- The most common imaging abnormality in patients with HTLV-I myelopathy is the presence of multifocal enhancing lesions in the spinal cord: less often, increased signal intensity in seen in brain white matter.

- The greatest risk factor for HTLV-I myelopathy is living in an area endemic for virus infection. Other sources of infection are blood transfusion, sexual contact, and intravenous drug abuse.

Further Reading

Osame M, Matsumoto M, Usuku K, Izumo S, Ijichi N, Amitani H, Tara M, Igata A. Chronic progressive myelopathy associated with elevated antibodies to human T-lymphotropic virus type I and adult T-cell leukemia-like cells. *Ann Neurol* *21*:117-122, 1987.

Bhigjee AI, Wiley CA, Wachsman W, Amenomori T, Pirie D, Bill PL, Windsor I. HTLV-I-associated myelopathy: clinicopathologic correlation with localization of provirus to spinal cord. *Neurology* *41*:1990-1992, 1991.

Herpes Simplex Virus-2 Meningitis

A 37-year-old woman develops fever, chills, and photophobia along with acute occipital headache and neck pain. She describes the headache as the "worst of my life." On examination, she is febrile and has nuchal rigidity. Small blister-like lesions are present on her lower back. Further history reveals that for the past 4 years, she has noted crops of vesicles on an erythematous base on various areas of her skin every 3-4 months. The lesions are not associated with systemic or neurological symptoms, and there is no history of genital herpes. A brain CT scan is normal. The CSF contains 345 WBCs, 96 percent mononuclear; the CSF protein is 150 mg percent, and glucose is 56 mg percent. CSF is sent for PCR for herpes simplex virus (HSV) DNA.

What do you do now?

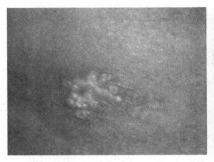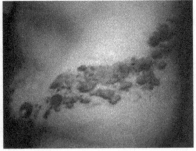

FIGURE 16-1 HSV-2 skin lesions. Note patchy skin lesions caused by HSV-2 (left), unlike the dermatomal-distribution lesions caused by VZV (right).

Multiple clinical features point to the diagnosis of aseptic meningitis, most likely produced by a virus. The specific agent that caused meningitis is suggested by recurrent patchy skin lesions characteristic of type 2 herpes simplex virus (HSV-2), even in the absence of a history of genital herpes. The patchy lesions caused by HSV-2 differ from the dermatomal-distribution lesions caused by VZV (Fig. 16-1). Thus, PCR of CSF with HSV-1- and -2-specific primers was requested. Only HSV-2 DNA was amplified, thus confirming the diagnosis of HSV-2 meningitis. The patient was treated with intravenous acyclovir for 5 days followed by oral valacyclovir for 2 weeks. She improved clinically, although 1 week later, the CSF still contained 307 WBCs, all mononuclear, with a CFS protein of 78 mg percent and glucose 51 mg percent.

HSV-2, a neurotropic DNA virus, is one of eight human herpesviruses. Primary infection may be asymptomatic or lead to genital herpes. Virus becomes latent in sacral ganglia. Reactivation produces genital herpes, or patchy vesicular skin lesions, or radicular pain with or without meningitis, all of which may recur. Thus, as listed in Table 16-1, clues to the diagnosis of HSV-2 infection are: (1) a history of recurrent meningitis, (2) a history of genital herpes; (3) recurrent patchy (zosteriform) skin lesions with neuropathy (e.g., sciatica); and (4) recurrent patchy skin eruptions with no history of neuropathy or genital herpes, but with meningitis, as in the case presented here.

Importantly, HSV-2 is the most common cause of benign recurrent lymphocytic meningitis. The term "Mollaret's meningitis" has no practical

TABLE 16-1   Clues to Diagnosis of HSV-2 Meningitis.

recurrent meningitis

concurrent or history of genital herpes

recurrent skin lesions with neuropathy

recurrent zosteriform eruptions

clinical or scientific use, and the name should be abandoned. If recurrent meningitis is bacterial, there may be communication between the outside world and the patient's CSF, perhaps due to a break in the cribriform plate of the ethmoid bone or at other sites. In that case, a radiologist should be enlisted to introduce a molecule such as radiolabeled indium into the CSF followed by imaging to identify the site of entry of bacteria.

Before the advent of antiviral agents against human herpesviruses, patients with recurrent HSV-2 meningitis recovered spontaneously. Today, patients with HSV-2 meningitis are routinely treated with antiviral agents, although it is not known how long patients should be treated, or whether intravenous antiviral therapy is superior to oral antiviral agents, or even whether antiviral treatment is beneficial. Brain imaging is normal in HSV-2 meningitis. For an accurate diagnosis of HSV-2 meningitis, the clinician must have a high index of suspicion and carefully review the patient's history for previous episodes of meningitis, recurrent skin lesions, genital herpes, and intermittent radicular symptoms. A careful examination of the entire skin will identify any active HSV-2 skin lesions.

KEY POINTS TO REMEMBER

- HSV-2 meningitis develops in patients with a history of genital herpes, recurrent patchy (zosteriform) skin eruptions, and/or recurrent radiculopathy.
- HSV-2 is the primary cause of recurrent meningitis.

Further Reading
Slavin HB, Ferguson JJ, Jr. Zoster-like eruptions caused by the virus of herpes simplex. *Am J Med* 8:456-467, 1950.

Craig CP, Nahmias AJ. Different patterns of neurologic involvement with herpes simplex virus types 1 and 2: isolation of herpes simplex virus type 2 from the buffy coat of two adults with meningitis. *J Infect Dis 127*:365–372, 1973.

Gonzales N, Tyler KL, Gilden DH. Recurrent dermatomal vesicular skin lesions: clue to diagnosis of herpes simplex virus 2 meningitis. *Arch Neurol 60*:868–869, 2003.

HIV Vacuolar Myelopathy

A 45-year-old man with AIDS develops fatigue, diarrhea, and weight loss and complains of leg weakness and tightness. In the past few months, he also experienced uncomfortable tingling in his toes. There is a history of primary syphilis treated with intramuscular penicillin and weekend binge-drinking, but no intravenous drug use. There is no family history of neurologic disease. He was diagnosed with AIDS 8 months ago. A few months ago, he was treated for *Pneumocystis carinii* pneumonia. Neurologic examination reveals cognitive slowing with impaired concentration and difficulty performing calculations. Cranial nerves are normal. Motor examination is normal in the arms, but there is a mild spastic paraparesis in the legs. DTRs are normal in the arms, increased at the knees, and absent at the ankles. The plantar responses are equivocal. The sensory examination reveals mildly decreased vibratory and proprioceptive sensation in the legs; pain sensation is intact. Serum vitamin B12, vitamin E, and folic acid levels are normal. A brain CT shows diffuse atrophy. The CSF is acellular; CSF protein is 68 mg percent, and VDRL is negative. PCR of the CSF for varicella zoster virus (VZV) and cytomegalovirus (CMV) DNA is negative.

What do you do now?

The site of disease must be established first. In this instance, the loss of epicritic sensory modalities with preservation of pain indicates disease in the posterior columns of the spinal cord, although a large-fiber neuropathy could also produce this type of dissociated sensory loss. The spasticity, weakness, and lack of a good plantar flexor response collectively indicate long tract disease. Posterior and lateral column disease is seen with vitamin B12, vitamin E, and folic acid deficiency, but those levels were normal in this patient. Familial spinocerebellar ataxia may also produce these signs, but there is no family history of neurological disease and no clinical features of kyphoscoliosis, high arched feet, or cardiac conduction defect as seen in patients with Friedreich's ataxia.

The development of posterior and lateral column disease in an HIV+ patient indicates HIV vacuolar myelopathy, the most common cause of spinal cord disease in AIDS patients.

Vacuolar myelopathy may present at any stage of HIV disease. Myelopathy develops insidiously. Leg weakness and tightness as well as dysesthesias are common. Urinary urgency and frequency are often early symptoms, as is erectile dysfunction. The examination usually reveals a spastic paraparesis, with loss of vibratory and proprioceptive sensation and a positive Romberg's sign. Pain and temperature sensation are usually preserved unless there is superimposed peripheral neuropathy. The CSF may be acellular or reveal a mild pleocytosis. More than 30 WBCs in the CSF should raise suspicion of other disorders such as neurosyphilis, tuberculous, VZV, or CMV myelitis.

Autopsy of patients with HIV vacuolar myelopathy reveals a high prevalence of pathologic involvement of the posterior and lateral columns in spinal cord white matter, while clinicopathologic correlations show that only 27 percent of these patients have symptoms and signs of myelopathy before death. Another retrospective study in AIDS patients with pathologic evidence of vacuolar myelopathy resembling subacute combined degeneration found dementia in a significant number of patients (as in this patient), as well as a high incidence of opportunistic infections, such as *Pneumocystis*, fungal infections, *Mycobacteria*, and even Kaposi's sarcoma. The high incidence of opportunistic infections suggests an association between the development of vacuolar myelopathy and the extent of immunosuppression.

Vacuolar myelopathy does not appear to be due to direct infection of the spinal cord, but is more likely the result of a metabolic disorder induced by viral or immunologic factors. Most HIV is found in macrophages, but not in neurons, and there does not appear to be a direct relationship between the presence of HIV and the development of myelopathy. Similarly, there is no correlation between the presence and severity of myelopathy and CSF levels of HIV RNA or tumor necrosis factor-α.

There is no definitive treatment for vacuolar myelopathy, and no controlled studies exist on the effect of highly active antiretroviral therapy (HAART) on the clinical manifestations of this disease. Despite serious illness, most patients with HIV myelopathy have normal serum vitamin B12 levels, and vitamin B12 supplements do not alter the course of disease.

Finally, evidence against the diagnosis of vacuolar myelopathy includes rapidly progressive myelopathy over days or weeks, the presence of a discrete sensory level, a CSF pleocytosis >30 cells, and back pain, any of which should signal the need for further testing to determine the cause of spinal cord disease.

KEY POINTS TO REMEMBER

- The clinical features of HIV vacuolar myelopathy are long tract signs with proprioceptive and vibratory loss.
- Patients suspected to have vacuolar myelopathy should be tested for serum vitamin B12, vitamin E, and folic acid levels.
- Patients with HIV vacuolar myelopathy have a high incidence of previous opportunistic infections and often some degree of cognitive impairment.

Further Reading

Petito CK, Navia BA, Cho ES, Jordan BD, George DC, Price RW. Vacuolar myelopathy pathologically resembling subacute combined degeneration in patients with AIDS. *N Engl J Med 312*:874–879, 1985.

Dal Pan GJ, Glass JD, McArthur JC. Clinicopathologic correlations of HIV-1-associated vacuolar myelopathy: an autopsy-based case-control study. *Neurology 44*:2159–2164, 1994.

18 Progressive Multifocal Leukoencephalopathy

A 51-year-old HIV+ man developed weakness of the left side of the face and left hand 4 months ago. In the past month, he has had increasing memory problems and got lost driving home. One month earlier, his CD4 T-cell count was 150. Neurological examination reveals impaired short-term memory. When told the positions of the hands on a clock, he cannot tell the right time. He is unable to spell "world" backward. Cranial nerves are normal. He has a mild spastic left hemiparesis and slight stereoanesthesia in the left hand. Other sensory modalities and coordination are normal. DTRs are a 3+ on the left side with a left extensor plantar response. A brain MRI reveals multifocal, asymmetric, and confluent subcortical nonenhancing white matter hyperintensities extending to the cortical gray matter (Fig. 18-1). CSF is clear, with normal opening pressure. CSF contains 8 WBCs, all mononuclear; CSF protein is 45 mg percent, and CSF glucose is normal. There are no oligoclonal bands, and CSF IgG is 8 percent (normal 3–13 percent) of total protein. PCR reveals amplifiable JC virus DNA.

What do you do now?

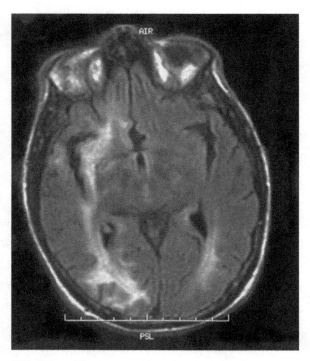

FIGURE 18-1 PML. Note multifocal, asymmetric confluent subcortical nonenhancing hyperintensities in the white matter that extend to the cortical gray matter.

The patient has the classic clinical, imaging, and virologic features of progressive multifocal leukoencephalopathy (PML), a demyelinating disease of the CNS that occurs predominately in severely immunosuppressed individuals. Before the HIV epidemic, PML was a rare disease seen only in patients with hematological malignancies, in organ transplant recipients, and in some patients with chronic inflammatory diseases. The prevalence of PML in the general population was estimated to be 4.4 cases per million individuals, but has now increased substantially; up to 5 percent of patients with AIDS develop the disease. Recently, immunomodulatory medications have emerged as a new group of drugs associated with development of PML, including natalizumab used for multiple sclerosis and Crohn's disease, rituximab for lupus, and efalizumab for psoriasis. The cause of PML is JC virus (JCV), a ubiquitous and exclusively human neurotropic DNA virus. Most adults are seropositive for JCV. JCV, a member of the highly oncogenic polyomavirus genus, is the only virus proven to cause demyelinating disease in humans. Virus in brain is found primarily in oligodendroctyes and to a far lesser extent in astrocytes.

PML typically presents with focal weakness (hemiparesis or hemianopia), cognitive dysfunction, and, less often, aphasia and coordination and gait difficulties. Disease does not usually involve the optic nerves or spinal cord. Interestingly, a recent study reported seizures in 16 of 89 patients with PML, a surprising finding because seizures are thought to arise from involvement of gray matter, whereas PML is a white-matter disease. Brain lesions are readily detected by MRI in the white matter and do not correspond to vascular territories. MRI lesions are hyperintense on T2-weighting and hypointense on T1-weighting; lesions do not enhance.

The diagnosis of PML is firmly established by detection of JCV DNA in CSF. There is no specific antiviral drug against JCV. A randomized controlled clinical trial of antiretroviral therapy alone or with intravenous or intrathecal cytarabine in 57 HIV+ patients with PML did not reveal any survival benefit in any treatment group. The current treatment goal in HIV+ patients with PML is restoration of the host adaptive immune response to JCV, a goal best reached by treatment with HAART drugs. Since the introduction of HAART, the median survival time of patients with PML has increased from 0.4 years to 1.8 years; some patients live as long as 60 to 188 months, most of whom had undetectable amounts of HIV in plasma and a mean CD4 T-cell count of 389, sufficient for protection against most opportunistic infections. In HIV- patients with PML, the main objective is to relax immunosuppression regimes and thereby enable the adaptive immune system to control infection. Unfortunately, decreasing these drugs in organ transplant recipients increases the risk of graft rejection. Although a cellular immune response directed against JCV is beneficial, rapid recovery of the immune system is not always favorable and can trigger an immune reconstitution inflammatory syndrome. Immune reconstitution is inferred based on worsening of the clinical state along with an increase in T-lymphocyte counts, usually after initiation of HAART therapy in HIV+ patients or after stopping immunosuppressive drugs in HIV- patients. Finally, a few novel clinical disorders caused by JCV include infection of cerebellar and cortical pyramidal neurons.

- PML usually presents with focal deficit or cognitive changes.
- PML most commonly occurs in HIV+ or AIDS patients, but also occurs in immunosuppressed patients with cancer or organ transplants and, most recently, in patients treated with natalizumab, efalizumab, and rituximab.
- JCV, the cause of PML, is a ubiquitous exclusively human virus, and the only virus proven to cause demyelinating disease in humans.
- MRI changes in PML are characterized by multifocal bilateral, asymmetric confluent white-matter lesions that do not enhance.
- Restoration of the host adaptive immune response to JCV in HIV+ patients by treatment with HAART drugs improves survival by months to years.

Future Reading

Tan CS, Koralnik IJ. Progressive multifocal leukoencephalopathy and other disorders caused by JC virus: clinical features and pathogenesis. *Lancet Neurol* 9:427–437, 2010.

Postherpetic Neuralgia

A 77-year-old woman develops left T6-distribution zoster and is treated immediately with valacyclovir, 1 gm 3 times daily for 7 days. She is also started on pregabalin, gradually titrated up to a dose of 50 mg 3 times daily. Unfortunately, 4 months later, she still has sharp, lancinating pain on the left chest below her breast. She guards the left chest from spray when she showers and wears loose-fitting clothes because her skin over the affected area is exquisitely sensitive to touch.

What do you do now?

Virtually all physicians who see patients with acute herpes zoster recognize pain that persists for more than 3 months as postherpetic neuralgia (PHN). PHN is common, with chronic pain after zoster estimated to occur in 20 percent to more than 40 percent of people over age 60. Few conditions in medicine are as challenging for the patient and the doctor. Individuals vary in their response to opioids and other analgesics, and the doctor must be prepared to work closely with the patient to determine an optimal regimen of treatment.

Like the patient herein, PHN patients are likely to have been taking some analgesic medication since the onset of zoster. Currently, the most commonly used drugs are gabapentin and pregabalin. A double-blind, placebo-controlled clinical trial found that pregabalin, 150 to 300 mg daily, reduced pain scores by more than 50 percent in patients with PHN. The mechanism of action and side-effect profile are similar to those of gabapentin. However, since pregabalin has a linear pharmacokinetic profile, there is less interindividual variability and the dose range is more narrow and predictable. Pregabalin may also have fewer side effects than gabapentin.

TOPICAL ANESTHETICS

Assuming a favorable but incomplete response to pregabalin in the PHN patient, a local anesthetic such as topical lidocaine-prilocaine cream or a patch of 5 percent lidocaine, 12 hr on and 12 hr off, should be considered. There are no significant side effects. Patches can be used alone or combined with pregabalin (my first choice of oral drug).

Capsaicin 0.075 percent cream can also decrease pain. Note that pain might be temporarily increased when beginning, presumably due to depletion of substance P or activation of nociceptors. A serious limitation of topical capsaicin cream is that it can burn the skin.

ANTICONVULSANTS

Both carbamazepine and phenytoin have been used with some success. I prefer carbamazepine. Remember that the patient is elderly, and the dose of drug should be small initially and increased gradually. The starting dose is 100 mg daily, increasing by an additional 100 mg every 3–4 days up to a dose of 600 mg (sometimes more). Side effects include drowsiness, unsteadiness, confusion, and constipation; carbamazepine may also cause a profound hyponatremia. Other anticonvulsants that reduce neuropathic pain (topiramate, lamotrigine, levetiracetam, zonegram, tiagabine, and lacosamide) may be helpful in PHN.

TRICYCLIC ANTIDEPRESSANTS

Among the tricyclic antidepressants, amitriptyline is the most extensively studied. In a double-blind, placebo-controlled clinical study, amitriptyline provided significant pain relief in patients with PHN. Unfortunately, the anticholinergic properties of tricyclics, particularly in the elderly, may cause dose-limiting side effects. Side effects (dry mouth, impotence, constipation, urinary retention, tachycardia, confusion) may be ameliorated by starting at low doses followed by slow titration and night administration when possible. The starting dose is 10 to 20 mg and, because of potential somnolence and sedation, it should be given at bedtime. This side effect may be of help in patients with insomnia, a common comorbidity in chronic pain patients. On occasion, doses of 100 to 150 mg per day may be necessary. When dosing above 75 to 100 mg per day (or lower if side effects are observed), blood levels should be determined to avoid toxicity. Desipramine, a tricyclic with less severe anticholinergic effects, and nortriptyline have also been shown to be effective in controlled studies to treat PHN. Remember that it takes several weeks to achieve maximum benefit from any antidepressant drug.

OPIOIDS

Depending on the intensity of the pain, opioids can be used early to treat both herpes zoster and PHN. A placebo-controlled clinical study with the extended form of oxycodone indicated significant pain relief in patients with PHN. The patient must always be alerted to potential side effects, including physical dependence, constipation, nausea/vomiting, sedation, and the possibility of addiction. Follow guidelines that do not allow patients to change dosing on their own. Only one practitioner writes the prescription, only one pharmacy is used, and the patient should be followed closely. Due to its low cost and long half-life, methadone (dolophine hydrochloride)

5–10 mg can be used to treat chronic pain. Regardless of the drug combination selected by the physician, a small dose of valium (~2 mg) taken a few times daily together with either pregabalin, antidepressants, or anticonvulsants often has a remarkable added effect.

Finally, antiviral therapy should be considered, in light of sizable evidence from clinical-virological correlations in patients with PHN, zoster sine herpete, and preherpetic neuralgia suggesting that chronic pain reflects active viral ganglionitis. Ongoing productive infection is likely to perturb neurons, resulting in continued pain. One study that used intravenous acyclovir followed by oral antiviral agents to treat patients with PHN months after onset showed a statistically significant reduction in pain in 53 percent of patients. While the study was not double-blinded or placebo-controlled, it did suggest the benefit of antivirals in patients with PHN. I recommend intravenous acyclovir for 10–15 days, although at present, insurance will not cover the cost of treatment. After intravenous treatment, I also recommend valacyclovir, 1 gm 3 times daily for a few months, with analgesia as recommended above.

Remember that although many zoster patients experience PHN for months to years, time is on the side of the patient and physician; there is a natural spontaneous resolution of PHN over time.

KEY POINTS TO REMEMBER

- No single best treatment for PHN is known. Both topical and systemic therapies can be initiated simultaneously. If pain is intense, opioids can be initiated early.
- Although the literature is not conclusive, it is recommended that herpes zoster infection be aggressively treated with antiviral agents to decrease PHN.

Further Reading

Gilden DH, Cohrs RJ, Mahalingam R. VZV vasculopathy and postherpetic neuralgia: progress and perspective on antiviral therapy. *Neurology* 64:21-25, 2005.

Cruciani R, Jabati S. Herpes zoster and postherpetic neuralgia. In: *Current Therapy in Neurologic Disease*, 7th edition (Johnson RT, Griffin JW, McArthur JC, eds). Philadelphia, PA: Mosby Elsevier, Chap 4, 84-86, 2006.

Quan D, Hammack BN, Kittelson J, Gilden DH. Improvement of postherpetic neuralgia after treatment with intravenous acyclovir followed by oral valacyclovir. *Arch Neurol* 63:940-942, 2006.

Bacterial, Spirochetal, Protozoan, and Prion Disorders of the Nervous System

20 Listeria Rhombencephalitis

A 28-year-old women developed sudden onset of severe vertigo, nausea, and vomiting. Her symptoms were exacerbated by head movement. By the fifth day of illness, she could not walk without assistance. She complained of right ear pain, a sore throat, and dull frontal headache. She denied nasal congestion, cough, tinnitus, hearing loss, or any visual changes. Temperature was 38.1°C. There were no skin lesions. The neurologic examination revealed a normal mental status. Visual fields were full, ocular motility was normal, and pupils were of equal size and reacted to light and accommodation. There was nystagmus on right gaze, left conjugate gaze paresis, and weakness of abduction looking to the right, hypalgesia on the right side of the face, intention tremor of the right arm and severe gait ataxia. The next day left peripheral facial weakness was noted, and her temperature was 38.4°C. On the 11th day of illness, her temperature was 38.4°C. There was nuchal rigidity. The CSF opening pressure was 244 mm H_2O, and the CSF contained 980 WBCs, 71 percent neutrophils; CSF protein was 93 mg percent, and glucose was 36 mg percent (blood glucose was 108 mg percent). CBC was normal, except for 71 percent neutrophils in the WBC count of the 6,800 cells per mm³. Gram stain revealed no organisms. CSF was sent for bacterial culture. A T2-weighted brain MRI FLAIR scan revealed a hyperintense signal in the brainstem (Fig. 20-1). A presumptive diagnosis of bacterial meningitis was made, and the patient was started on intravenous ampicillin and ceftriaxone.

What do you do now?

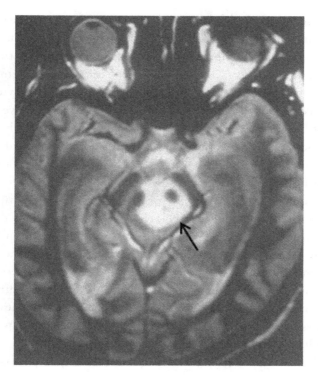

FIGURE 20-1 Listeria monocytogenes rhombencephalitis. T2-weighted FLAIR MRI show hyperintense signal in the brainstem (arrow).

The patient's clinical features of fever, stiff neck, and profound CSF pleocytosis indicate meningitis. Because most of the CSF cells were neutrophils and the CSF glucose was low, the patient needs to be started on antibiotics immediately while awaiting the results of CSF culture. Importantly, there were multiple signs indicating involvement of lower cranial nerves, which along with a gait ataxia pointed to the pons as the primary site of disease, confirmed by brain MRI. A bacterium with a predilection for the lower brain stem is *Listeria monocytogenes*, a gram positive rod.

On the third hospital day, CSF culture isolated *Listeria*. While Listeria rhombencephalitis develops most commonly in healthy and immunocompetent individuals, remember that Listeria also develops in patients in the extremes of life, the very young and elderly, in alcoholics, and in immunocompromised individuals such as organ transplant recipients and patients taking steroids. A biphasic clinical pattern is common with a prodromal phase of headache, fever, and leukocytosis and the subsequent development of pontomedullary cranial nerve paresis. Cases of Listeria have been described in which high protein levels lead to obstruction of CSF pathways and the development of hydrocephalus. Listeria is virtually never seen on the initial gram stain, but can be cultured from CSF, blood, and other organs, such as liver if microabscesses are present. *Listeria monocytogenes* is sensitive to multiple antibiotics, such as ampicillin and chloramphenicol. Sometimes the brain stem (pontobulbar) encephalitis occurs without meningitis and thus is designated as rhombencephalitis. As in this case, it is best to start antibiotic treatment with the assumption that the meningitis is bacterial, while awaiting confirmation from culture. A delay in instituting treatment for bacterial meningitis is more likely to be detrimental to the patient than a few days of intensive antibiotic treatment, which can be stopped later when culture is negative.

In adults with bacterial meningitis, the major pathogens are *Haemophilus influenzae*, *Neisseria meningitidis*, *Streptococcus pneumoniae*, and *Listeria monocytogenes*. Importantly, gram negative organisms account for 30–40 percent of nosocomial (hospital-acquired) meningitis with the major factors being neurosurgery (craniotomy) and head trauma (basal skull fracture) as well as neurosurgical devices (deep brain stimulation, ventriculoperitoneal shunt, cochlear implants) or a CSF leak. The organisms seen in infected craniotomies are often *Staphlococcus aureus* or various gram negative organisms. Device-related meningitis is typically associated with coagulase negative staph, propionabacterium acnes, and other indolent gram positive rods, such as bacillus species. Postneurosurgical meningitis includes gram positive organisms such as *Staphylococcus aureus*, strep species, and coagulase negative staphylococcus. Gram negative organisms account for about 40 percent of bacterial meningitis and include pseudomonas, acinetobacter, *Klebsiella pneumoniae*, and enterobacter species.

- Bacterial meningitis must always be treated immediately, while awaiting results of gram stain and culture.
- *Listeria monocytogenes* has a predilection for the brain stem and may present exclusively as pontobulbar encephalitis.
- Listeria meningitis is seen most often in newborns but also in the elderly and immunocompromised populations.

Future Reading

Durand ML, Calderwood SB, Weber DJ, Miller SI, Southwick FS, Caviness VS Jr, Swartz MN. Acute bacterial meningitis in adults. A review of 493 episodes. *N Engl J Med.* 1993 Jan *328*:21-28, 1993.

A 25-year-old man develops personality and behavioral changes that evolve over 4 months. He is easily angered, withdrawn, and expresses suicidal thoughts. His speech and walking become slower. In the past week, he becomes mute. On the day of hospital admission, he stops using his right side. A scaly maculopapular rash is seen on the soles of his feet (Fig. 21-1). On neurologic examination, he is alert and corporative. His muteness fluctuates, and, when he does speak, a nonfluent aphasia is evident. He has right central facial weakness and a spastic paraparesis, greater on the right. Pinprick sensation is decreased on the right. DTRs are hyperactive in all extremities, and there is sustained clonus at both ankles with bilateral Babinski signs. His gait is wide-based and spastic. A brain MRI scan reveals extensive white matter hyperintensities bilaterally (Fig. 21-2). The CSF opening pressure is normal. The CSF is clear and contains 110 WBCs, 98 percent mononuclear; CSF protein is 109 mg percent, glucose is 55 mg percent, and there are 15 oligoclonal bands.

What do you do now?

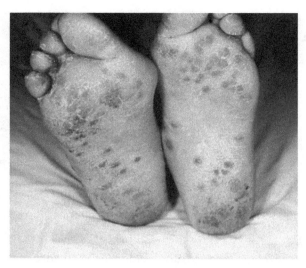

FIGURE 21-1 Skin rash in neurosyphilis. Multiple nonpruritic, well-circumscribed, scale-covered, maculopapular erythematous plaques are seen over the soles of the feet. (From Brinar VV, Habek M. Dementia and white-matter demyelination in young patient with neurosyphilis. *Lancet 368*(9554):2258; 2006. Reprinted with permission from Elsevier Limited.)

The patient has chronic meningoencephalitis with focal neurologic deficit. This combination of features is characteristic of granulomatous meningoencephalitis. Diagnostic considerations must include tuberculous and fungal meningitis, CNS sarcoid, Lyme disease, and neurosyphilis. A maculopapular scaly rash on the palms of the hands and soles of the feet is often seen in neurosyphilis, and in conjunction with the neurologic symptoms and signs, makes meningovascular syphilis the leading diagnosis. A positive CSF VDRL confirms the diagnosis.

Meningovascular syphilis is one of many forms of neurosyphilis, all of which are caused by the spirochete *Treponema pallidum*. Spirochetes, which are bacteria with double membranes, and mostly long and helically coiled, are distinguished from other bacteria by the location of their flagella, sometimes called axial filaments that run lengthwise between the inner and outer bacterial membrane. Most spirochetes are free-living and anaerobic. A different spirochete (*Borrelia burgdorferi*) causes Lyme disease (see Chapter 26). Meningovascular syphilis occurs anywhere from 3 months to 10 years after primary infection. Often the genital ulcerative lesion (chancre) has been forgotten, and many patients do not have a history of skin rash at the time of presentation. The CSF usually contains a lymphocytic pleocytosis with increased protein and oligoclonal bands. Arterial involvement produces focal narrowing as seen in other vasculitides. Vascular involvement may result in extensive white matter disease (Fig. 21-2) that mimics multiple sclerosis or a leukoencephalopathy.

In addition to headache, fever, stiff neck, and focal deficit, patients with meningovascular syphilis also become demented and develop cerebral atrophy, indicating overlap with general paresis (dementia paralytica), which is characterized by severe dementia along with weakness, tremor of the hands and tongue, pupillary abnormalities, and loss of bladder and bowel control, usually 10 to 20 years after primary infection. Another form of neurosyphilis is tabes dorsalis, which results from inflammation of the posterior roots and subsequent atrophy of the dorsal horns of the spinal cord, and is

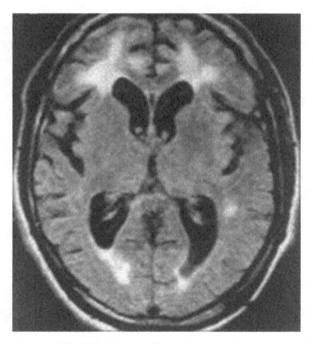

FIGURE 21-2 Neurosyphilis. T2-FLAIR brain MRI reveals white matter hyperintensities at the border of white and gray matter. Note also moderately severe cortical atrophy.

characterized by optic atrophy, shooting pains, a wide-based gait, severe loss of position and vibratory sensation, including deep pain sensation, Argyll Robertson pupils (small irregular pupils that exhibit light-near dissociation), impaired sphincter function, and Charcot joints. Neurosyphilis may also present with isolated optic atrophy, the reason that all patients with monocular visual loss should have a serologic test for syphilis. If any other form of neurosyphilis is strongly suspected and the CSF VDRL is negative, an FTA-ABS test should be performed.

Neurosyphilis is treated with high doses of aqueous penicillin G intravenously for 10 to 14 days. Clinical improvement is accompanied by resolution of the CSF pleocytosis and loss of VDRL positivity in the CSF. Today, many patients with neurosyphilis are HIV+ or have AIDS. Because these patients are immunocompromised, close clinical and CSF examinations are needed after treatment.

KEY POINTS TO REMEMBER

- Meningovascular syphilis may present with headache, fever, and stiff neck (meningitis) in combination with focal deficit (stroke) and cognitive impairment.
- Brain imaging in meningovascular syphilis may reveal meningeal enhancement and focal ischemic lesions.

Further Reading

Marra CM. Neurosyphilis. In: *Central Nervous System Infectious Diseases and Therapy* (Roos KL, ed). New York: Marcel Dekker, 237–252, 1997.

Brinar VV, Habek M. Dementia and white-matter demyelination in a young patient with neurosyphilis. *Lancet 368*:2258, 2006.

22 Tuberculous Meningoencephalitis

A 38-year-old man complains of lethargy and intermittent confusion for the past 6 weeks. Last week, he developed double vision, worse when looking to the right. His wife reports that he occasionally forgets appointments and cannot remember recent events. His temperature is 101°F. The neurological examination reveals that he is oriented to time, place, and person, and his knowledge of current events is adequate. He does well in making similarities and comparisons. He has difficulty concentrating. There is short-term memory loss. When asked to name the months of the year backward, he does so accurately but slowly. When given the positions of the large and small hands on a clock, he makes mistakes in telling the exact time. He cannot repeat five numbers backward. The cranial nerve examination reveals an inability to abduct the right eye fully. There is left-sided ptosis, and the left pupil is larger than the right and reacts sluggishly to light. The remainder of the cranial nerves and funduscopic examination are normal. There is a mild spastic right hemiparesis. All sensory modalities are intact. DTRs are brisk, slightly greater on the right, without any pathological reflexes. Gait is slightly wide-based, and he has difficulty standing on either foot alone. Brain

MRI scan reveals T2 hyperintensities (Fig. 22-1, arrows) consistent with infarction. Angiography demonstrates multifocal areas of arterial narrowing at the base of the brain (Fig. 22-2, arrows). CSF examination reveals an opening pressure of 320 mm. The CSF is cloudy and contains 240 WBCs, 86 percent mononuclear. CSF protein is 280 mg percent, and glucose is 40 mg percent. CSF is sent for gram stain, smear for acid-fast bacilli, serology, Lyme titer, cryptococcal antigen, bacterial and fungal culture, cytology, and angiotensin-converting enzyme (ACE) levels.

What do you do now?

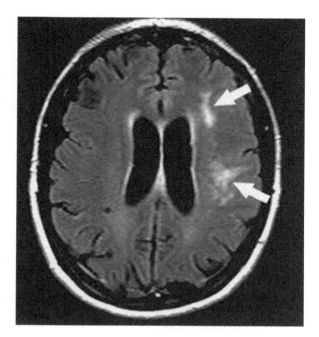

FIGURE 22-1 Tuberculous meningoencephalitis. Brain MRI reveals white-matter hyperintensities consistent with infarction in the left hemisphere (arrows) and enlarged ventricles. (From Renard D, Morales R, Heroum C. Tuberculous meningovasculitis. *Neurology* 68(20):1745; 2007. Reprinted with permission from Wolters Kluwer Health.)

The clinical features indicate meningoencephalitis and stroke. Inflammatory and infectious diseases to consider are meningovascular syphilis, Lyme disease, sarcoidosis, tuberculous and fungal meningitis, and multifocal varicella zoster virus vasculopathy. CNS lymphoma can also produce this clinical picture.

While awaiting test results, the patient was started on 4-drug standard therapy for tuberculous meningitis. Serology, Lyme titer, a search for cryptococcal antigen, cytology, and ACE levels were all normal. On the 3rd hospital day, a positive smear for acid-fast bacilli was reported, clinching the diagnosis of tuberculous meningitis. A 7-day course of steroids was added to the patient's treatment regimen. Involvement of the 6th and 3rd cranial nerves, as seen in this patient, is common in tuberculous meningitis. The classic CSF abnormalities in tuberculous meningitis are an elevated opening

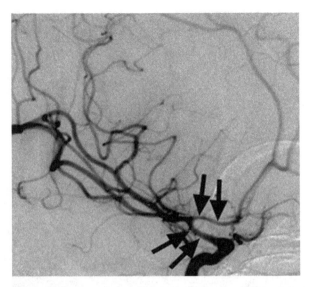

FIGURE 22-2 Angiography shows multifocal arterial narrowing at the base of the brain. (From Renard D, Morales R, Heroum C. Tuberculous meningovasculitis. *Neurology 68*(20):1745; 2007. Reprinted with permission from Wolters Kluwer Health.)

pressure and high WBC count with a predominance of mononuclear cells and a low glucose. Areas of multifocal infarction as well as arterial narrowing at the base of the brain are also common in tuberculous meningitis. The MRI may also show leptomeningeal enhancement, enlarged ventricles, and prominent ring-enhancing lesions throughout the brain (Fig. 22-3, arrows).

Tuberculous meningitis is a serious condition. Death often occurs in 6–8 weeks in patients who are not diagnosed and treated immediately. However, disease can also last for months. In addition to acid-fast stain and culture, PCR is now also being used to detect *Mycobacterium tuberculosis* DNA.

KEY POINTS TO REMEMBER

- Like other subacute to chronic meningoencephalitides (syphilis, fungal infections, and sarcoidosis), *Mycobacterium tuberculosis* causes meningitis and stroke.

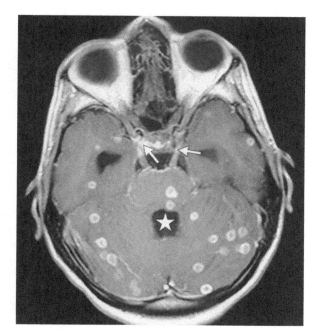

FIGURE 22-3 Brain MRI demonstrates multiple T1 contrast-enhancing intracranial tuberculomas, ventricular enlargement (star), and leptomeningeal enhancement at the base of the brain (arrows). (From Akhaddar A, Boucetta M. Images in clinical medicine: multiple intracranial tuberculomas. *N Engl J Med 365*(16):1527; 2011. Reprinted with permission from the Massachusetts Medical Society.)

- The 3rd and 6th cranial nerves are commonly involved in tuberculous meningitis.
- Characteristic MRI changes in tuberculous meningitis include leptomeningeal enhancement, particularly at the base of the brain, as well as focal ischemic lesions and tuberculomas.

Further Reading

Verdon R, Chevret S, Laissy JP, Wolff M. Tuberculous meningitis in adults: review of 48 cases. *Clin Infect Dis 22*:982, 1996.

Margado C, Ruivo N. Imaging meningo-encephalic tuberculosis. *Eur J Radiol 55*:188-192, 2005.

23 Raeder's Paratrigeminal Syndrome

A 51-year-old woman experiences intermittent sensations of right ear fullness and vertigo for 3 months. In the past week, she developed right-sided otitis media, right facial numbness, stabbing headaches, and intermittent drooping of the right eyelid. Examination reveals an incomplete Horner's syndrome (right-sided ptosis and miosis without anhidrosis) and right-sided trigeminal-distribution hypalgesia. A CT angiogram shows no evidence of carotid artery dissection. A contrast-enhanced T1-weighted MRI reveals a complex fluid collection and opacification in the mastoid air cells (Fig. 23-1A), consistent with mastoiditis that extends to the area around the internal carotid artery. Blood cultures are negative. The CSF is normal.

What do you do now?

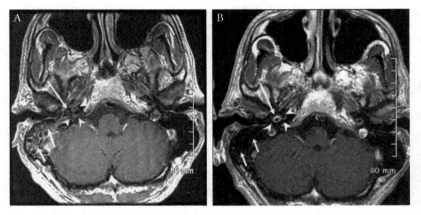

FIGURE 23-1 Raeder's paratrigeminal syndrome. During acute disease, a contrast-enhanced T1-weighted MRI reveals heterogeneous enhancement mixed with a low T1 signal in the mastoid air cells and around the carotid artery, consistent with inflammation (A). Three months after antibiotic therapy, there is near complete resolution of inflammatory changes in the mastoid air cells in the temporal bone around the carotid artery (B). Long arrows point to the carotid artery, short arrows point to mastoid air cells, and arrowheads indicate areas around the carotid artery.

The patient has a painful Horner's syndrome with trigeminal nerve involvement. This is known as Raeder's paratrigeminal syndrome. Raeder's syndrome has diverse etiologies. The causes in most instances are intrinsic carotid artery disease, such as aneurysm, dissection, or stenosis, none of which were indicated by angiography. The protracted history, development of otitis media with fluid collection and opacification in mastoid air cells consistent with mastoiditis and extending to the area around the internal carotid artery indicate that chronic inflammation was the cause of Raeder's syndrome in the patient. She was treated with intravenous vancomycin and oral piperacillin/tazobactam for 3 days followed by oral doxycycline and levofloxacin for 5 weeks. Three months later, her headaches and trigeminal-distribution hypalgesia had resolved, although a partial Horner's syndrome was still evident, perhaps due to permanent damage to sympathetic nerve fibers around the carotid artery. Brain imaging revealed near-complete resolution of inflammation in the mastoid air cells and around the carotid artery (Fig. 23-1B).

Although Horner originally described features of involvement of the cervical sympathetic nerves in 1869, Raeder recognized that Horner's syndrome may result from a lesion anywhere along the course of these sympathetic fibers, and that the extent of the syndrome varied with the location of the lesions. For example, in this patient, the absence of anhidrosis reflects the path of the sympathetic fibers for sweat along the external carotid artery, whereas the fibers controlling the dilator papillae and superior palpebral muscle follow the internal carotid. Raeder also reported the relationship between "paralysis of the oculopupillary sympathetic nerves and pain in the trigeminal nerve distribution, implicating the paratrigeminal area of the middle fossa of the cranium." Recognition that periarterial inflammation can cause Raeder's syndrome should alert the clinician to the need for relevant imaging studies.

KEY POINTS TO REMEMBER

- Raeder's syndrome is characterized by trigeminal nerve involvement and a painful Horner's syndrome.
- Raeder's syndrome may be due to intrinsic disease of the carotid artery (aneurysm, dissection, or stenosis) or infectious/ inflammatory disease that has extended from the middle ear to the area around the carotid artery.
- Patients with Raeder's syndrome should have vascular imaging to rule out disease of the carotid artery as well as brain MRI to look for disease in mastoid air cells or sinus and to visualize the area around the carotid artery.
- Patients with Raeder's syndrome due to infectious/inflammatory disease may have a favorable response to antibiotics.

Further Reading

Grimson BS, Thompson HS. Raeder's syndrome: a clinical review. *Surv Ophthalmol* 24:199-210, 1980.

Nagel MA, Bert RJ, Gilden D. Raeder's syndrome produced by extension of chronic inflammation to the internal carotid artery. *Neurology* 79:1296-1297, 2012.

A 47-year-old pregnant woman from Panama develops progressively increasing frontal headache and unsteadiness. Except for a slightly wide-based gait and the inability to hop on either foot, she displays nothing remarkable on neurological and funduscopic examination. A contrast-enhanced brain MRI is normal. During the course of her hospitalization, four CSF examinations are performed. The CSF opening pressure is always normal and the CSF is clear. Each CSF sample contains many RBCs and WBCs, with a pleocytosis consisting of both neutrophils and mononuclear cells, elevated protein and decreasing glucose values (Table 24-1). CSF from the 4th tap is centrifuged, and the pellet is cultured for acid-fast bacilli and fungi. Chest X-ray reveals old granulomatous disease. Cryptococcal antigen, angiotensin-converting enzyme levels, Lyme titers, VDRL, PCR of CSF for varicella zoster virus (VZV) DNA, and serology for anti-VZV antibody are all negative. She is treated with antituberculous therapy, but her headache worsens and she becomes intermittently confused.

What do you do now?

TABLE 24-1 **Serial CSF Findings**

	RBCs	WBCs	% neutrophils	% mononuclear	protein mg%	glucose mg%
1	80	208	48	52	126	45
2	75	190	42	58	142	35
3	41	111	61	39	138	28
*4	64	148	35	65	180	10

* high-volume tap

The clinical features and CSF findings indicate chronic meningitis. The old granulomas on chest X-ray are consistent with tuberculous or fungal infection. The presence of pleocytosis consisting of abundant neutrophils, mononuclear cells, and RBCs on repeated CSF exams are a clue to etiological diagnosis. Remember that RBCs are rarely seen in tuberculous meningitis. Furthermore, their presence should not be attributed to a "bloody tap" since RBCs in CSF that do not decrease from tubes 1 to 4 are found in chronic CNS infectious disorders caused by fungi, VZV, and cytomegalovirus (CMV).

On the 20th hospital day, a fungus identified as *Histoplasma capsulatum* was isolated from the CSF. Fungi are eukaryotic organisms such as yeasts, molds, and the more familiar mushrooms, and are distinguished from plants, animals, and bacteria by the presence of chitin in the cell walls. Although culture was successful in this case, it is often difficult to isolate a fungus from CSF. Other studies that help in diagnosing chronic tuberculous or fungal meningitis involve a high-volume CSF tap (approximately 50 ml), which should then be centrifuged and the pellet cultured for fungi. Remember that like many viruses, fungi are cell-associated, and the chances of isolating a fungal agent increase when more cells are provided to the microbiology lab.

Most fungal meningitis is encountered in immunosuppressed patients. *Cryptococcus, Candida,* and *Aspergillosis* infection are the most common causes of fungal meningitis in immunocompromised individuals. If cryptococcal antigen is present, the diagnosis of Cryptococcal meningitis is confirmed. The armamentarium of antifungal drugs has expanded from only amphotericin decades ago. See the "Further Reading" section below for optimal drug, route, dose, and length of treatment.

Finally, remember that the clinical picture of chronic meningitis and focal neurologic deficit is characteristic of tuberculous, fungal, and lymphomatous meningitis; Lyme disease; neurosyphilis; and sarcoidosis.

KEY POINTS TO REMEMBER

- Fungi usually seed at the base of the brain and propagate in arteries. The combination of chronic basilar meningitis and stroke is characteristic of fungal meningitis.
- In patients with subacute to chronic meningitis, consider tuberculosis, fungi, syphilis, sarcoidosis, lymphoma, VZV, and CMV as causative agents.
- Of the infectious agents that cause chronic meningitis, only fungi, VZV, and CMV produce RBCs in the CSF.

Further Reading

Gilden D, Miller EM, Johnson WG. Central nervous system histoplasmosis after rhinoplasty. *Neurology 24*:874-877, 1974.

Davis LE, Porter BS. Fungal infections. In: *Current Therapy in Neurologic Disease*, 7th edition (Johnson RT, Griffin JW, McArthur JC, eds). Philadelphia, PA: Mosby Elsevier, Chap 7, 161, 2006.

Whipple's Disease

A 50-year-old man is hospitalized for evaluation of
ophthalmoplegia and dementia. Two years earlier,
he developed double-vision followed weeks later
by easy fatigability and hypersomnia. One year
ago, he experienced profuse night sweats, shoulder
arthralgias, and mild headache, all of which responded
to anti-inflammatory agents. One month ago, he
developed diarrhea, low-grade fever, and rectal bleeding.
Endoscopy reveals punctate esophagitis with scattered
erosions in the stomach. Gastrointestinal biopsy
specimens show atypical macrophage infiltrates and no
malignancy. Neurologic examination indicates severe
memory impairment, and he makes numerous mistakes
when trying to repeat 5 numbers backward. He cannot
look down and has limited up-gaze. There is an upper
motor neuron pattern of weakness in the right arm and
leg, but no other neurological signs. The CSF opening
pressure is normal, and the CSF is acellular; CSF protein
is 60 mg percent. A serological test for syphilis is
negative. CSF and serum angiotensin-converting enzyme
(ACE) levels are normal. Brain MRI reveals hyperintense
lesions in the hypothalamus and medial temporal lobe
(Fig. 25-1).

What do you do now?

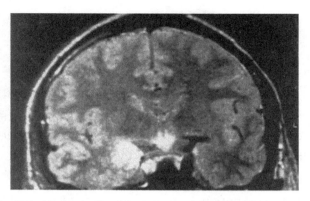

FIGURE 25-1 Whipple's disease. T2-weighted MRI scan demonstrates hyperintense lesions in the hypothalamus and superomedial region of the temporal lobe.

The patient developed a progressive neurologic disorder of 2 years' duration. He also had fever and autonomic nervous system involvement, as indicated by hypersomnia and possibly by night sweats. Importantly, he had progressive dementia and ophthalmoplegia, primarily vertical, indicating disease rostral to the collicular plate. The MRI revealed hyperintense lesions in the hypothalamus and the medial temporal lobe.

Degenerative, neoplastic, inflammatory, and nutritional disorders must all be considered. The patient's clinical course was too rapid for progressive supranuclear palsy, and the focal lesions seen on imaging would not be expected in any of the Parkinson-plus syndromes, such as Shy-Drager, striatonigral degeneration, and other mixed motor system disorders. The clinical history and the neurological exam do not rule out glioma, lymphoma, or sarcoma. Wernicke's syndrome is unlikely because the patient was neither an alcoholic nor nutritionally deficient. Chronic inflammatory disorders such as tuberculous, sarcoid, and fungal infections and syphilis deserve consideration; however, tuberculous meningitis is unlikely to last for 2 years, and the patient did not have the CSF pleocytosis expected with tuberculous meningitis, CNS sarcoidosis, or syphilis. Furthermore, the negative serology and normal ACE levels make syphilis and sarcoidosis even less likely. A chronic angiitis is also a possibility, but the patient did not have severe headache or even a modest CSF pleocytosis. A paraneoplastic syndrome seems unlikely, since disease progressed for 2 years without development of a systemic tumor and since the hypothalamus is not usually involved in limbic encephalitis.

Importantly, the patient had arthralgias and gastrointestinal disease in combination with dementia and vertical ophthalmoplegia, a combination that is characteristic of Whipple's disease. Whipple's most commonly affects the gastrointestinal tract and joints, and macrophages filled with periodic acid-Schiff-positive material are seen. In the brain, Whipple's disease has a predilection for the hypothalamus, hippocampus, and periaqueductal gray matter. The neurologic picture is usually characterized by dementia, vertical ophthalmoplegia, and myoclonus. Oculomasticatory myorhythmia (vertical oscillations of the eyes with concurrent contractions of the masticatory muscles) occurs only in Whipple's disease, although many patients, including the patient described here, did not display that. Whipple's disease should always be considered when brain imaging reveals involvement of the hypothalamus, the high brain stem, and medial temporal lobe, particularly if lesions enhance. Arthralgias, abdominal pain, fever, diarrhea, malabsorption, and weight loss are common.

Whipple's disease is caused by the bacillus *Tropheryma whipplei*. PCR has high sensitivity and specificity for the bacillus, and the CSF in this patient was found to contain *Tropheryma whipplei* DNA. After treatment with trimethoprim-sulfamethoxazole for 6 months, the patient showed no progression of neurological or systemic disease, although severe memory loss and vertical gaze palsy remained.

KEY POINTS TO REMEMBER

- The main clinical features of Whipple's disease are dementia, ophthalmoplegia (usually vertical), and myoclonus.
- Whipple's disease has a predilection for the high brain stem, hypothalamus, and medial temporal lobe, usually seen as increased signal on brain MRI.
- Whipple's disease affects not only the gastrointestinal tract and joints but also the CNS.
- Laboratory diagnosis is best confirmed by PCR amplification of *Tropheryma whipplei* DNA from CSF.

Further Reading

Gilden DH, Kleinschmidt-Demasters BK. A 47-year-old man with ophthalmoplegia and dementia. *J Neuroimag 1*:140–145, 1991.

Fenollar F, Puéchal X, Raoult D. Whipple's disease. *NEJM 356*:55–66, 2007.

26 Lyme Disease

A 20-year-old man was hospitalized because of intermittent fever of 3 weeks duration and recent onset of facial diplegia. Two weeks ago, he developed headache, and his temperature was 100°C. His headache subsided, but fever continued. Four days before admission, he developed a pruritic rash on his waist and over his knees. Three days ago, he developed discomfort in his neck that gradually worsened along with numbness and weakness in his right hand. The patient was a graduate student and had been in good health. He drank alcohol socially and had no history of drug abuse or sexually transmitted diseases. Two months earlier, he went camping in northern New York State, where he was bitten by flies. Six weeks ago, he had a weekend vacation in Nantucket. He had no history of joint pains, tick bites, or exposure to tuberculosis. No one in his family had a similar illness.

On admission, he appeared alert but uncomfortable and had pain in his neck and right arm. Blood pressure and vital signs were normal. A desquamating erythematous rash was observed on his abdomen and knees (Fig. 26-1). There was slight tenderness to palpation over the left orbit and globe. Visual fields and acuity were normal, although there was mild blurring of the nasal margins of both optic disks. He had nystagmus when looking laterally in either direction. He was unable to wrinkle his forehead, close his eyes tightly, frown, smile, or retract the angles of his mouth on either side. Hyperacusis to loud sounds was observed. Taste was absent on the right half of the tongue. His speech was fluent, but his voice was hoarse. The remainder of the cranial nerves were normal. Motor function revealed normal tone and strength, except for slight weakness of hand grip on the right; all sensory modalities were normal. DTRs were 3+ in the legs and 2+ in the arms, and both plantar responses were flexor.

CBC was normal, except that 76 percent of his WBCs were neutrophils. The sedimentation rate was normal, and blood chemistries and a urine analysis were normal. A T1-weighted contrast-enhanced MRI scan of the brain and neck revealed leptomeningeal enhancement at the base of the brainstem (Fig. 26-2) and in multiple areas of the cervical spine, particularly at C5-6 on the right; in the brain, multiple areas of increased signal intensity were also present in white matter and periventricular regions. Two CSF exams were performed on the 1st and 7th hospital day. CSF opening pressures were normal, and the CSF was clear on both occasions. On day one, the CSF contained 453 WBCs, 97 percent mononuclear; on day 7, there were 375 cells, 99 percent mononuclear. CSF protein was markedly elevated, and CSF glucose was normal both times. Gram stain and acid-fast stain were negative, culture for bacteria and fungi, test for cryptococcal antigen, and serology were negative. Angiotensin-converting enzyme (ACE) levels were normal. PCR did not amplify herpes simplex virus or varicella zoster virus DNA. There was no anti–West Nile virus IgM antibody. Serum and CSF were sent for an Epstein-Barr virus antibody panel, as well as for Lyme antibody and Rocky Mountain spotted fever antibody.

What do you do now?

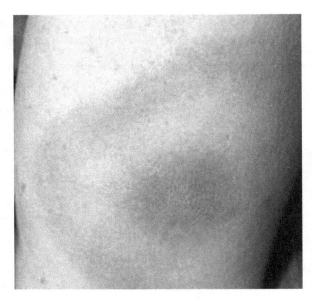

FIGURE 26-1 Lyme disease. Erythematous rash with "target" appearance on the leg of a patient with Lyme disease.

The patient presents with meningoradicular symptoms and signs including facial nerve involvement bilaterally and a CSF pleocytosis. In patients with chronic meningoencephalitis, tuberculosis, fungal meningitis, sarcoidosis, syphilis, and Lyme disease must be ruled out. Peripheral facial weakness (unilateral or bilateral) is not a feature of tuberculous meningitis (TB has a predilection for cranial nerves III and VI), fungal meningitis, or neurosyphilis, but is seen in sarcoidosis and Lyme disease. As an aside, other disorders that exhibit bilateral facial weakness are lymphoma and various forms of GBS. There is no rash in tuberculous or fungal meningitis. The fact that the patient was not immunocompromised also makes fungal infection less likely, and a negative test for cryptococcal antigen and culture for fungi further helped to rule out fungal infection. The absence of a positive acid-fast stain or culture for acid-fast bacilli along with normal ACE levels and a negative serology make tuberculous meningitis, neurosyphilis, and CNS sarcoidosis less likely. With rickettsial infection (scrub typhus, Rocky Mountain spotted fever), patients with CNS involvement usually have more prominent brain abnormalities, such as seizures and cloudy consciousness.

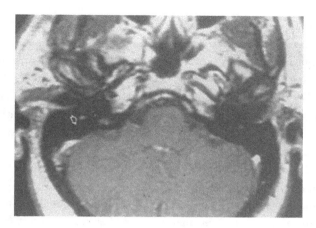

FIGURE 26-2 T1-weighted brain MRI at the level of the brainstem shows enhancement in the right 7th cranial nerve (arrowhead).

The rash of typhus begins centrally and spreads peripherally, while that of Rocky Mountain spotted fever starts peripherally and usually becomes petechial. Neither of those rashes is pruritic, as was this patient's rash.

Importantly, there was a history of arthralgias and rash that preceded the onset of neurological disease. Arthralgias are common in Lyme disease, and more than half of all Lyme disease patients with neurological disease have a history of rash weeks earlier. One week after admission, serological studies revealed antibody to *Borrelia burgdorferi* in serum and CSF, which confirmed the diagnosis of Lyme disease.

Lyme disease, a multisystem illness that affects the skin, nervous system, heart, and joints, is caused by the tick-borne spirochete *Borrelia burgdorferi*. *Borrelia burgdorferi* can be found in CSF and synovial joint fluid.

The Lyme disease spirochete is transmitted by two species of Ixodes ticks. The principal hosts for ticks are mice and deer, although Ixodes ticks have been found in multiple types of wild animals and many species of birds. Although the patient does not remember being bitten by a tick, he was in an area of New England where ticks are endemic. Tick bites when remembered are generally one to 2 weeks before the early features of malaise, fatigue, fever, myalgia, arthralgia, sore throat, abdominal pain, and regional adenopathy that often accompany the rash. The rash in Lyme disease, erythema migrans, is an expanding erythematous lesion that occurs at the site of the tick bite approximately 1 to 2 weeks after infection. It begins as a macule and enlarges over a week to form an annular erythematous plaque often with a characteristic central area, giving a "target" appearance. Although rash may be pruritic or painful, it is most often asymptomatic. While erythema migrans has been considered to be the only pathognomonic criterion to diagnose Lyme disease, only 60 to 80 percent of patients ever develop or notice it at the onset of infection.

About 15 to 20 percent of patients in the United States with Lyme disease develop frank neurologic involvement. Stiff neck and cranial neuropathies usually follow rash. Facial palsy can be the only neurologic manifestations of Lyme disease, even without meningitis. Other cranial nerves frequently involved are III, IV, and VI. Overall, the cardinal neurological findings of Lyme disease are: lymphocytic meningitis, cranial neuropathies (with the VII nerve being most commonly affected, often bilaterally), and painful radiculitis. Patients may also experience peripheral neuropathy presenting as radiculopathy, plexopathy, or a diffuse polyneuropathy, often mimicking GBS. White matter lesions can also be seen in Lyme disease. Numerous ocular disorders also occur in Lyme disease including follicular conjunctivitis, keratitis, intraocular inflammation, orbital inflammation, pupillary abnormalities, and optic nerve dysfunction.

Multiple antibiotics have been used to treat Lyme disease. After months of treatment with ceftriaxone and doxycycline, the patient made a full recovery.

KEY POINTS TO REMEMBER

- The skin rash of Lyme disease often has a "target" appearance.
- Neurologic manifestations of Lyme disease are chronic and present most often as meningoencephalitis, cranial nerve palsies (with the 7th nerve being most often involved and often bilaterally) and painful radiculitis.
- Imagining abnormalities in Lyme disease include meningeal enhancement as well as bilateral deep-seated and periventricular lesions mimicking demyelinating disease.
- Confirmation of Lyme disease is provided by detection of antibody to *Borrelia burgdorferi* in serum and/or CSF.

Further Reading

Logigian EL, Kaplan RF, Steere AC. Chronic neurologic manifestations of Lyme disease. *N Engl J Med 323*:1438-1444, 1990.

Steere AC. Lyme disease. *N Engl J Med 345*:115-125, 2001.

27 CNS Toxoplasmosis

A 46-year-old man with AIDS is hospitalized for progressive visual loss in the right eye and multiple focal seizures on the day of admission. In the past 1–2 months, he noted deteriorating vision in the right eye as well as double vision, increased by gaze in any direction. Seizures always begin with weakness in the right hand; seconds later, the hand tingles, after which tonic-clonic movements develop in the right arm followed by rhythmic jerking of the entire right side. Episodes are brief and without loss of consciousness. The interictal neurologic examination reveals lethargy and decreased emotional response. In the past 17 months, he had an episode of herpes zoster and most recently pneumocystis pneumonia. Examination reveals chemosis and proptosis on the right. Visual acuity is 20/60 OD and 20/20 OS. Funduscopic examination reveals optic disk swelling, macular edema, and retinal hemorrhages, consistent with central retinal vein occlusion. The neurologic examination indicates an intact mental status and a mild spastic right hemiparesis. MRI brain scan with orbital cuts shows proptosis of the right eye with inflammation of the eyelid, chorioretinal thickening, a thickened optic nerve sheath and central focus of enhancement in the optic nerve (Fig. 27-1A); in the left hemisphere, a T1-weighted MRI showed a hypointense ring-enhancing mass with a mural nodule and some surrounding edema (Fig. 27-1B). Collagen vascular disease studies, a 4-vessel cerebral angiogram, and CSF are normal. CSF cytology and serology were negative. Serum and CSF were sent for Lyme and Toxoplasma antibody titers.

What do you do now?

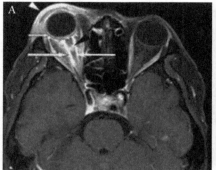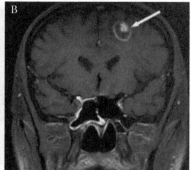

FIGURE 27-1 CNS toxoplasmosis. Brain MRI with orbital cuts. (A) In the right eye, note tram track enhancement along thickened optic nerve sheath on both sides of the optic nerve (long arrows) and a central focus of optic nerve enhancement (black arrowhead), a thickened sclera and chorioretinal complex (short arrow) with proptosis and contrast-enhanced thickening of the right eyelid (white arrowhead). (B) Contrast-enhanced T1-weighted MRI reveals a hypointense ring-enhancing mass with a mural nodule and some surrounding edema.

The patient presents with both ocular and cerebral disease. The ocular problem includes proptosis, chorioretinal and optic nerve disease, and central retinal vein occlusion. The cerebral disorder was characterized by a hypointense lesion surrounded by a ring-enhancing capsule and edema. While multiple organisms can produce such an abscess, the combination of orbital disease and a cerebral abscess, particularly in an AIDS patient, should signal the likelihood of toxoplasmosis. No Lyme antibody was detected in serum or CSF. Toxoplasma antibody titers were 1:1024 in serum and 1:16 in CSF.

Toxoplasmas are protozoans, that is, eukaryotic, often motile organisms. Toxoplasmosis encephalitis is the most common cause of brain abscess in HIV-infected patients, often occurring when CD4+ cell counts are less than 100. Clinical features of toxoplasmosis, particularly in immunocompromised patients, are subacute to chronic encephalitis manifesting as confusion, delirium, obtundation, and coma, occasionally accompanied by focal and generalized seizures as well as focal deficit. Lesions produced by *Toxoplasma gondii* are typically located at gray-white matter junctions as well as in deep white matter, thalamus, and basal ganglia. Most lesions enhance in a ringed, nodular or homogeneous pattern and are surrounded by edema. It is important to differentiate toxoplasmosis from lymphoma, as the latter benefits from radiation therapy. On T2-weighted MRI, lymphoma is usually isointense to hypointense relative to white matter, whereas toxoplasmosis is more likely to be hyperintense. Treatment includes sulfadiazine with pyrimethamine for 3 to 6 weeks. Remember that drug therapy targets actively growing tachyzoites, but has limited effects on slow-growing bradyzoites, thus recurrence is common.

KEY POINTS TO REMEMBER

- Toxoplasmosis is the most common cause of cerebral abscess in patients with AIDS.
- Toxoplasmosis infection of the eye and brain often occur together.
- In immunosuppressed patients, toxoplasmosis must be differentiated from other causes of focal disease, particularly lymphoma.
- Biopsy is reserved for patients who have no clinical or radiographic response after a week of therapy.

Future Reading

Horowitz SL, Bentson JR, Benson F, Davos I, Pressman B, Gottlieb MS. CNS toxoplasmosis in acquired immunodeficiency syndrome. *Arch Neurol 40*:649–652, 1983.

Tan IL, Smith BR, von Geldern G, Mateen FJ, McArthur JC. HIV-associated opportunistic infections of the CNS. *Lancet Neurol 11*:605–617, 2012.

A 41-year-old man is hospitalized for increasing episodes of frontal headache, nausea, and intermittent double vision. He moved to the United States from Mexico at age 18. He has had a seizure disorder since age 10 that was well-controlled with anticonvulsants. His wife reported that his memory is not what it used to be, and that he has difficulty remembering a grocery list or his placement of things around the house. He had a negative tuberculin skin test at another hospital. There is no history of syphilis or other sexually transmitted disease, gastrointestinal symptoms, problems with gait, or incontinence of bladder or bowels. He takes no medications other than anticonvulsants. The neurologic examination reveals memory loss. He is able to remember 2 of 3 cities, 1 of 3 numbers, and 3 of 5 objects in the room after 5 minutes. He cannot repeat 5 numbers backward. The remainder of the neurologic examination is normal. CBC and sedimentation rate are normal. Brain MRI reveals a large number of cysts of varying size, none of which enhance (Fig. 28-1). The CSF is clear and colorless, and the opening pressure is normal; CSF contains 30 WBCs, 95 percent mononuclear; CSF protein and glucose are normal. CSF culture for acid-fast bacilli and fungi, and a serologic test for syphilis and test for cryptococcal antigen are all negative.

What do you now?

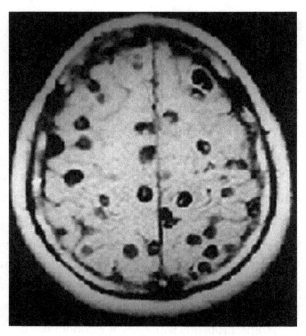

FIGURE 28-1 Cysticercosis. Note massive numbers of cysts resembling "Swiss cheese" in the brain of a patient with neurocysticercosis.

This patient with a long-standing seizure disorder is now experiencing headache, nausea, diplopia, and cognitive problems. While none of his symptoms is unique to any disease, they are all common in neurocysticercosis, a disorder revealed by brain MRI that showed the classic "Swiss cheese" appearance produced by multiple cysts of varying size. Furthermore, the patient grew up in Mexico, one of many countries where cysticercosis is endemic. Thus a diagnosis of neurocysticercosis is likely.

Worldwide, cysticercosis is the most common parasitic infection of the human CNS. Cysticercosis is caused by an infection with the pork tapeworm *Taenia solium*. Infection is acquired by ingesting insufficiently cooked pork containing tapeworm larva or by eating contaminated food prepared by a *Taenia solium* carrier with sticky tapeworm eggs under their fingernails. A tapeworm then develops in the intestines. The tapeworm causes few clinical symptoms but does release proglottids (segments of the tapeworm containing male and female reproductive organs) which pass into the stool, liberating viable ova or eggs. Stool examination may reveal ova of the pork tapeworm. Ova are also partially digested in the stomach and release oncospheres (larva of the tapeworm contained within the external embryonic envelope and armed with 6 hooks) that penetrate intestinal mucosa to reach the bloodstream. Oncospheres are distributed throughout the body, but have a predilection for the brain, where they lodge in small blood vessels between gray and white matter as well as in the meninges, ependyma, and choroid plexus. When alive, cysts evoke only a mild surrounding inflammatory reaction, consisting of eosinophils and giant cells with gliosis, which does not generally cause clinical symptoms, although patients may have seizures. Cysts typically remain viable for 2 to 6 years. Most patients have more than one cyst in the brain. The incubation period is long; symptoms often do not appear until many years after infection with the tapeworm. In many patients, the patient is asymptomatic until the cysts degenerate. To prevent development of the intestinal tapeworm, all pork should be thoroughly cooked before consumption; freezing pork at -20°C for several days will also inactivate cysticerci. Cooks should also be checked for cysticeral eggs on their hands and under their fingernails.

Neurocysticercosis occurs mainly in developing countries. Disease is endemic in Mexico, Latin America, South America, India, and China. The most common symptom of neurocysticercosis is seizures. Seizures are more often focal than generalized. Headache is also frequent, along with visual disturbances, nausea, abdominal cramps, diarrhea, and rarely psychiatric illness. If patients develop hydrocephalus, they may experience headache, unsteadiness when walking, and cognitive problems simultaneously. Cysticercosis should be suspected in patients who have lived in an endemic area and present with seizures, mental status changes, or symptoms and signs of acute or chronic increased intracranial pressure.

Both CT and MRI exhibit numerous diffusely distributed cystic areas that create a "Swiss cheese" appearance. On MRI, cysts are bright on T2-weighting. CT scanning is better at detecting small areas of calcification and is cheaper than MRI, a significant issue in Third-World countries. MRI is more sensitive in detecting small lesions, brain stem or intraventricular lesions, and perilesional edema around calcified lesions, and is better at visualizing the scolex and more useful in evaluating degenerative changes in the parasite. MRI is also superior to CT for follow-up of patients after therapy. Overall, a reasonable practical approach involves a CT scan followed by MRI in patients with inconclusive findings or with negative CT scans but in whom there is strong clinical suspicion of cysticercosis.

The CSF in neurocysticercosis is abnormal in about 50 percent of cases. A lymphocytic pleocytosis is most common. Importantly, eosinophils are seen in about 15 percent of patients. When a cyst leaks, peripheral eosinophilia may be pronounced.

Anticonvulsants are used to control seizures. Specific antihelminthic drugs include praziquantel, which effectively treats cysticercosis of the brain parenchyma. Albendazole is also effective in patients who had a poor response to praziquantel and is considerably less expensive. Acute destruction of parasites induced by treatment with praziquantel frequently induces adverse reactions through an inflammatory response and increased protein in the CSF, reactions that can be suppressed by corticosteroid therapy. There is insufficient data to conclude that albendazole is superior to praziquantel. Hydrocephalus develops in about 25 percent of patients with neurocysticercosis and is treated by ventriculoperitoneal shunting. Overall, the treatment of cysticercosis is highly individualized; factors used to tailor therapy include the location of the cysts, symptoms such as seizures or features of hydrocephalus, the viability of the cysts, and degree of the host inflammatory response. The patient described herein above was treated with albendazole, and his symptoms resolved, and he was of course maintained on anticonvulsants.

KEY POINTS TO REMEMBER

- Cysticercosis is the most common CNS parasite. Most cases in America are in immigrants from Mexico and Latin America.
- While tapeworm infection is acquired by eating undercooked pork containing larval cysts, neurocysticercosis is also transmitted by ingestion of contaminated food prepared by a *Taenia solium* carrier with sticky tapeworm eggs under their fingernails.
- Most patients with neurocysticercosis are asymptomatic.
- Seizures and headaches are the most common clinical feature of neurocysticercosis.

- Neurocysticercosis is usually diagnosed based on the demonstration of cysts on MRI or CT scan.
- Treatment of parenchymal cysts using albendazole with or without corticosteroids hastens their disappearance and reduces seizure recurrence. Management of extraparenchymal cysts in the meninges or ventricles is more difficult and often requires shunting.

Further Reading

García HH, Del Brutto OH. Imaging findings in neurocysticercosis. *Acta Trop 87*:71-78, 2003.

Davis LE. Do patients with neurocysticercosis benefit from cysticidal therapy? *Nat Clin Pract Neurol 3*:22-23, 2007.

Jakob-Creutzfeldt Disease

A 61-year-old man experiences rapidly progressive memory loss. He had been well until 3 months earlier, when he became forgetful, had trouble with word-finding and was intermittently confused. One month ago his walking became unsteady, and in the past week he has had difficulty standing, even with the aid of a walker. In the past few weeks, his voice has become soft, and he became withdrawn. He has not been exposed to any unusual chemicals or toxic materials. On examination he knows what city he is in, but does not know the date or the name of the president of the United States. He exhibits a childlike demeanor. Motor examination reveals a spastic quadriparesis. Cerebellar testing reveals severe clumsiness and dysmetria. Spontaneous movement of the arms and legs are occasionally accompanied by myoclonus. DTRs are brisk, but both plantar responses are flexor. There is a snout reflex and bilateral palmomental reflexes. His gait is "magnetic," as though his feet are glued to the floor, and he uses the wall for support when walking. An MRI reveals increased signal intensity in the putamen and globus pallidus (Fig. 29-1). The CSF opening pressure is normal, and the CSF is clear, with normal CSF protein and glucose. PCR does not reveal amplifiable JC virus DNA. An EEG shows generalized slow-wave activity. A CBC, liver and renal function studies, serology, search for thyroid antimicrosomal antibodies, and urine screen for drugs and heavy metals are all negative. Tests for syphilis, multiple antineuronal antibodies, antinuclear antibodies, rheumatoid factor, and antineutrophil cytoplasmic antibodies are negative.

What do you do now?

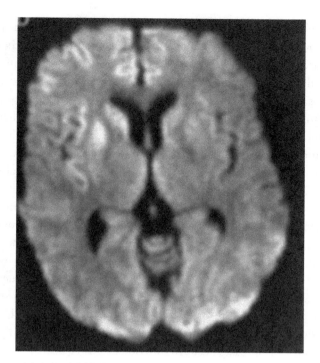

FIGURE 29-1 Jakob-Creutzfeldt disease. Diffusion-weighted MRI sequences in a patient with Jakob-Creutzfeldt disease shows increased signal in the right striatum, right frontal and insular cortex, and bilaterally in the occipital cortex. (From Tschampa HJ, Kallenberg K, Urbach H, Meissner B, Nicolay C, Kretzschmar HA, Knauth M, Zerr I. MRI in the diagnosis of sporadic Creutzfeldt-Jakob disease: a study on inter-observer agreement. *Brain 128*(Pt 9):2026-2033; 2005. Reprinted with permission from Oxford University Press.)

Rapidly progressive dementia with motor problems can certainly be seen with a tumor, particularly a butterfly glioma of the corpus callosum. Patients with diffuse vascular disease can also exhibit the same clinical features, but the course is too fast for a multi-infarct dementia. A normal brain MRI ruled out a tumor, multiple infarcts, or hydrocephalus. A normal CSF would not be expected if the patient had an infectious or inflammatory CNS disease. Metabolic disorders resulting in chronic end-stage liver or renal disease were quickly ruled out by normal serum chemistries. Hashimoto's thyroiditis may produce a profound rapidly progressive encephalopathy and diffuse background slowing on EEG, but there were no thyroid antimicrosomal antibodies. The lack of detectable mercury in urine ruled out Minamata disease, a disorder that killed Japanese fisherman in epidemic proportions years ago. There were no serum autoantibodies indicative of limbic encephalitis or a paraneoplastic syndrome. A normal sedimentation rate and the absence of antinuclear antibody, anti-double-stranded DNA antibodies, antiribonucleoprotein antibodies, and SS-A and SS-B antibodies make diffuse vasculitis unlikely. There was no history of chronic diarrhea or ophthalmoplegia, but the patient should still be tested for Whipple's disease by examining the CSF for amplifiable *Tropheryma whipplei* DNA.

Rapidly progressive dementia with widespread motor problems, a normal CSF, and deep-seated hyperintensities seen on MRI indicate the likelihood of Jakob-Creutzfeldt disease, one of the transmissible spongiform encephalopathies. Note that "Jakob" precedes "Creutzfeldt" because Jakob's original paper described dementia and upper motor neuron and extrapyramidal signs as well as myoclonus along with the pathology of spongiform encephalopathy, whereas not all of Creutzfeldt's original cases were spongiform encephalopathies. Dementia is the most common feature of Jakob-Creutzfeldt disease. Pyramidal and extrapyramidal signs are frequent. Myoclonus may also develop, usually late in many patients. Most cases occur in individuals 50–70 years old, although there is a report of disease in a 20-year-old woman. The typical course of Jakob-Creutzfeldt disease is less than 6 months, although some cases last for a few years.

The CSF is normal in patients with Jakob-Creutzfeldt disease. Detection of the 14-3-3 protein can be helpful, although its absence does not rule out Jakob-Creutzfeldt disease. Furthermore other rapidly progressive CNS diseases are associated with a positive 14-3-3 test. An EEG typically reveals diffuse slow waves as well as intermittent bursts of periodic discharges. Brain biopsy is performed only when diagnosis is unclear. Pathological changes include status spongiosus of the neuropil, widespread neuronal loss, and prominent astrocytosis.

About 85–90 percent of cases occur sporadically without any identifiable cause or exposure. The remainder is genetic in origin, caused by mutations that alter the amino acid sequence of the prion protein. Rarely, Jakob-Creutzfeldt disease has been transmitted by growth hormone, dura mater grafts, corneal transplantation, and cerebral electrodes, all contaminated with prions. Blood can theoretically transmit disease, but accidental transmission is highly unlikely; nevertheless blood and other body fluids should be handled cautiously.

Variant Jakob-Creutzfeldt disease due to ingestion of prion-contaminated beef or beef products occurs mostly in teens and young adults. The Gerstmann-Straussler-Scheinker syndrome is a familial form of Jakob-Creutzfeldt disease that presents with truncal and appendicular ataxia in addition to pyramidal and extrapyramidal signs. The cerebellum is predominately affected, and amyloid plaques are found in addition to classic spongiform encephalopathy. Another form of spongiform encephalopathy is familial fatal insomnia, which is characterized by weeks to months of intractable insomnia and dysfunction of the autonomic nervous system. Pathologic changes are localized primarily in the thalamus and inferior olivary nucleus.

Jakob-Creutzfeldt and Kuru were first shown to be transmissible by Gajdusek and Gibbs and later found to result from neuronal accumulation of a misfolded pathogenic isoform, designated PrP^{Sc}, of a normal brain protein known as prion protein (PrP^C). When PrP^{Sc} binds to endogenous PrP^C, the latter is converted to PrP^{Sc}. The Nobel Prize was awarded to Carlton Gajdusek, who showed that Jakob-Creutzfeldt disease is transmissible, and to Stanley Prusiner, who identified prions as the infectious material.

There is no specific treatment for Jakob-Creutzfeldt disease. Accumulating evidence supports a unifying role for prions in neurodegenerative diseases. In Alzheimer's disease, which is characterized by amyloid plaques, intracerebral inoculation of brain homogenates from Alzheimer's patients into marmosets led to the development of amyloid plaques, with incubation periods exceeding 3.5 years. This demonstrates that disease is transmissible and supports the existence of a disease-causing prion. Further, in the tauopathies, a group of neurodegenerative diseases characterized by tau protein aggregation, mutant tau has been shown to be transmissible in transgenic mice, with tau aggregates observed 1 year after inoculation. Finally, in Parkinson's disease, α-synuclein accumulates into Lewy bodies in neurons; Lewy bodies have been found in grafted fetal brain cells a decade after transplantation into Parkinson's patients, raising the possibility that α-synuclein proteins can also become prions that were synthesized in the grafted cells. The convergence of studies demonstrating prions in the pathogenesis of multiple neurodegenerative disease is exciting. The potential exists to identify prion ligands by positron-emission tomography long before symptoms appear. Treatment could be achieved with molecules that diminish precursor proteins, interfere with the conversion of precursors into prions, or enhance prion clearance.

KEY POINTS TO REMEMBER

- Jakob-Creutzfeldt disease is a rapidly progressive dementia associated with pyramidal and extrapyramidal signs, ataxia, and myoclonus.
- The CSF is normal in patients with Jakob-Creutzfeldt disease.
- The MRI in Jakob-Creutzfeldt disease is normal or may show hyperintense deep-seated signals, primarily in the basal ganglia and thalamus.
- It remains unclear how conventional Jakob-Creutzfeldt disease is acquired, but disease can be transmitted by intimate contact from contaminated corneal transplants, electrodes, growth hormone, and dura mater grafts.

Further Reading

Mastrianni JA. Prion diseases. *Clin Neurosci Res* 3:469–480, 2004.

Prusiner SB. Cell biology: a unifying role for prions in neurodegenerative disease. *Science* 336:1511–151, 2012.

Inflammatory Diseases of the Nervous System of Unknown Etiology

Acute Disseminated Encephalomyelitis

You are called to the emergency room to consult on a 20-year-old undergraduate student. The ER physician says that the man is not moving much and giggles inappropriately. He thinks the patient is hysterical or malingering, but wants a neurologist to "clear the air." The patient exhibits a flat affect and chuckles briefly 3–4 times during the time you take his history and examine him. He is cooperative, and his speech is clear and fluent. He has trouble with serial 7's and cannot spell "world" backward. He can repeat words, but cannot identify a "pen" or "finger" by name. Cranial nerves, muscle tone, strength, and sensation are intact. Finger-to-nose and heel-to-knee testing are smooth but slow. His gait is slow and cautious but not unsteady. Reflexes are brisk and symmetric, and there are bilateral extensor plantar responses. You recognize features of an encephalopathy that include a pseudobulbar palsy. You order a brain MRI scan, which reveals multiple small asymmetric white matter lesions, some of which enhance (Fig. 30-1). The CSF opening pressure is normal. The CSF is clear and contains 88 WBCs, all mononuclear; CSF protein is 47 mg percent, glucose is 100 mg percent, and there are no oligoclonal bands.

What do you do now?

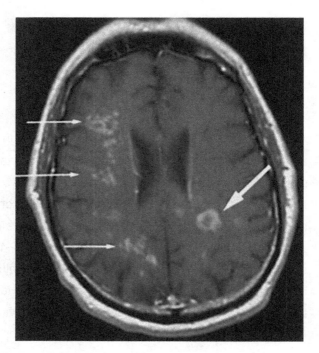

FIGURE 30-1 Acute disseminated encephalomyelitis. Contrast-enhanced T1-weighted MRI scan shows numerous small enhancing abnormalities (thin arrows) in the white matter. A larger ring-enhancing lesion (thick arrow) is seen in the left hemisphere. (From Ravin P, Hedley-Whyte ET. Case records of the Massachusetts General Hospital. Weekly clinicopathological exercises. Case 34-2002. A 55-year-old man with cognitive and sensorimotor findings and intracranial lesions. *N Engl J Med 347*(18):1433-1440; 2002. Reprinted with permission from the Massachusetts Medical Society.)

The patient developed acute onset neurologic disease, with spontaneous intermittent giggling, a flat affect, and impairment of higher cognitive function. The disinhibited behavior is characteristic of a pseudobulbar palsy which, even if it stood alone, indicates bilateral neurologic disease above the level of the brain stem, a notion supported by bilateral extensor plantar responses and confirmed by multiple asymmetric white matter lesions on MRI. The inexperienced clinician might interpret the spontaneous giggling as functional and not recognize the serious organic nature of the patient's disease. The CSF mononuclear pleocytosis indicates an inflammatory disorder. Taken together, the leading diagnosis is acute disseminated encephalomyelitis (ADEM). Other less likely considerations are a neoplastic process, granulomatous disease with chronic meningitis and multiple infarcts, and other forms of vasculitis.

The clinical features of ADEM include any combination of headache, mental status changes, depressed consciousness, seizures, focal motor deficit, and ataxia. A history of preceding respiratory or gastrointestinal symptoms may or may not be recalled. The CSF may be normal early, but hundreds of WBCs, predominantly mononuclear, are often seen later. MRI shows multifocal asymmetrical white matter lesions, many of which enhance. Disease evolves for many weeks.

Historically, disseminated encephalomyelitis was first described in patients who had received the Pasteur rabies vaccine containing brain tissue and later after smallpox immunization (postvaccinial encephalomyelitis). Before the days of measles vaccine, approximately 1 in 1,000 children who had measles developed demyelinating postinfectious encephalitis. Similarly, from 1 in 63 to 1 in 200,000 patients who had vaccinia (smallpox) developed postinfectious encephalomyelitis. Discontinuance of vaccination against smallpox and immunization of children against measles virus have eliminated these forms of demyelinating encephalomyelitis. Importantly, postinfectious encephalomyelitis, postvaccinial encephalomyelitis, ADEM, and experimental autoimmune encephalomyelitis (EAE) all show a lag between encounter with antigen and onset of a monophasic illness, and the pathological hallmarks of all are perivenular inflammation and demyelination.

Patients must be diagnosed quickly because early aggressive treatment with corticosteroids prevents permanent neurologic disease and death. Treatment should begin immediately with prednisone, no less than 1 mg/kg body weight daily for at least 6 weeks. Decades ago, clinical-pathological correlations of the natural history of ADEM revealed that disease progresses for more than a month, as evidenced by additional pathological findings that develop up to 30 days after the onset of symptoms as well as new MRI lesions that are seen as late as 6 weeks after the onset of disease (Fig. 30-2). All too often, I have consulted on a case of ADEM that has "relapsed," only to learn that the patient was successfully treated with steroids for 2 weeks but deteriorated when steroids were discontinued. Importantly, a monophasic episode of ADEM often lasts for about 6 weeks, approximately the same duration as an acute exacerbation of multiple sclerosis (MS). In distinguishing ADEM from a severe first episode of MS, remember that headaches,

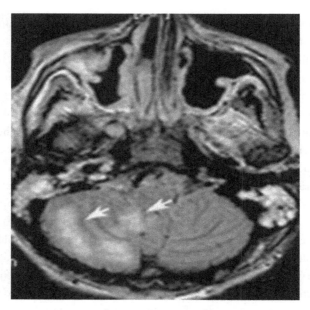

FIGURE 30-2 Multiple high signal lesions on T2-FLAIR MRI in the right cerebellar hemisphere 6 weeks after the onset of ADEM (arrows) that was not present at 3 weeks (not shown). (From Honkaniemi J, Dastidar P, Kähärä V, Haapasalo H. Delayed MR imaging changes in acute disseminated encephalomyelitis. *AJNR Am J Neuroradiol 22*(6):1117-1124; 2001. Reprinted with permission from American Society of Neuroradiology.)

seizures, and CSF cell counts over 80 are common in ADEM but not in MS. Oligoclonal bands are seen in both conditions but less often in ADEM. Patients who fail to respond to steroid treatment can sometimes be treated successfully with plasma exchange or intravenous immunoglobulin.

KEY POINTS TO REMEMBER

- ADEM is a monophasic demyelinating disorder of the CNS, characterized by headache, mental status changes, focal neurologic deficit, a CSF pleocytosis, and sometimes oligoclonal bands.
- In ADEM, white matter lesions on MRI are bilateral and asymmetrical and may enhance.

- Patients with ADEM should be treated with high-dose corticosteroids for at least 6 weeks before tapering drug, since "relapses" are often due to premature discontinuance of drug therapy.

Further Reading

Carpenter S, Lampert PW. Postinfectious perivenous encephalitis and acute hemorrhagic leukoencephalitis. In: *Pathology of the Nervous System* (Minckler J, ed). New York: McGraw-Hill, Vol. 3, Chap 168, 2260-2268, 1972.

Caldemeyer KS, Smith RR, Harris TM, Edwards MK. MRI in acute disseminated encephalomyelitis. *Neuroradiology 36*:216-220, 1994.

Behcet's Disease

A 35-year-old woman with a past history of recurrent ulcers around the mouth and genitalia comes to see you urgently because of headache, double vision, and unsteadiness. She reports intermittent pain and swelling of the wrists and ankle joints. Her temperature is 101.4° F. Ulcers are present in her mouth and on the vulva. She is alert, oriented, and anxious. She giggles briefly multiple times. Her fundi appear normal. She has a left-gaze paresis, right central facial weakness, a right hemiparesis, right-sided hypalgesia, dysarthria, and an ataxic gait. The jaw jerk and DTRs are hyperactive, greater on the right, and both plantar responses are extensor. A T2-weighted MRI scan reveals multiple high-intensity lesions in deep cerebral white matter and the pons, none of which are periventricular. The CSF contains 35 WBCs, all mononuclear; the CSF protein is 65 mg percent, and glucose and cytology are normal. There is no PCR-amplifiable DNA of herpes simplex virus, varicella zoster virus, or *Tropheryma whipplei* in the CSF. The sedimentation rate is high, and elevated fibrin split products are found in serum. A serological test for syphilis is negative, and there are no HIV or Lyme antibodies. Serum and CSF levels of angiotensin-converting enzyme are normal. Serum

HLA-B5 is positive. A 25-gauge needle is inserted into the skin of the forearm, and a 2- to 3-mm papule is seen over the area the next day. A mouth mucosal biopsy reveals no inclusions, and PCR is negative for HSV DNA.

What do you do now?

During the history, the patient's spontaneous intermittent giggling suggested a pseudobulbar palsy, indicative of bilateral upper motor neuron disease above the level of pons and further manifest by dysarthria and bilateral long tract signs. The MRI revealed multiple deep-seated and brain stem lesions, and the CSF revealed an inflammatory condition. The most common causes of such conditions include granulomatous disease (tuberculosis, fungal infection, syphilis, or sarcoidosis), Lyme disease, lymphoma, and rarely Whipple's disease.

The presence of nonherpetic recurrent mucocutaneous ulcers, particularly in a patient who later develops neurologic disease, suggests Behcet's disease, a multisystem inflammatory disease. Although any organ can be involved, there is enhanced vulnerability of the eye (uveitis and retinal vasculitis), nervous system (meningoencephalitis, venous sinus thrombosis, and focal parenchymal disease preferentially affecting deep-seated structures and the brain stem), and skin (erythema nodosum). Mucocutaneous lesions usually precede disease in the eye and nervous system. The CSF is usually inflammatory, but can be acellular. If there is venous sinus thrombosis (Fig. 31-1), the CSF opening pressure may be high.

Other features commonly seen in Behcet's and present in this patient are an elevated sedimentation rate, increased fibrin split products, positive HLA-B5, and a positive pathergy test (development of a papular lesion 24–48 hours after insertion of a needle into the skin). The patient did not have eye involvement, but painless intermittent loss of vision is common. The conjunctiva may be injected, and a hypopyon (leukocytic exudate) may be seen in the anterior chamber (Fig. 31-2). Pathologically, small veins are infiltrated by lymphocytes and plasma cells.

Behcet's disease is known as Silk Route disease because it is common in Turkey, Iran, Iraq, India, Pakistan, China, Korea, and Japan. The cause is unknown. Corticosteroids are used to treat neurological disease, although rigorous proof of their effectiveness is wanting. Immunosuppressive drugs have also been used. A recent report of a favorable response with infliximab monotherapy in a long-standing case resistant to conventional therapy requires confirmation.

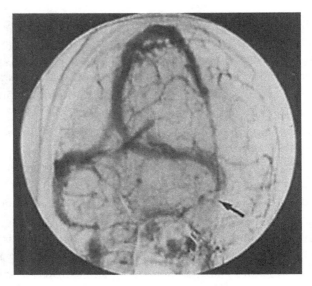

FIGURE 31-1 Venous digital subtraction angiogram demonstrating occlusion of the left sigmoid sinus (arrow) in a patient with Behcet's disease. (From Harper CM, O'Neil BP, O'Duffy JD, Forbes GS. Intracranial hypertension in Behcet's disease: demonstration of sinus occlusion with use of digital subtraction angiography. *Mayo Clin Proc 60*:419–422; 1985. Reprinted with permission from Elsevier.)

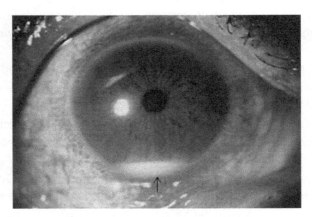

FIGURE 31-2 Conjunctival inflammation and a hypopyon (leukocytic exudate) in the anterior chamber (arrow) of the eye of a patient with Behcet's disease. (From Soloway S, Weissgold D. Images in clinical medicine: hypopyon. *N Engl J Med 334*(23):1512; 1996. Reprinted with permission from the Massachusetts Medical Society.)

KEY POINTS TO REMEMBER

- The diagnosis of Behcet's disease requires a history of recurrent mucocutaneous ulcers.
- Behcet's disease can affect any organ, but the nervous system, eye, and skin are most often involved.
- Behcet's disease may involve any part of the brain or spinal cord, although deep-seated structures in the brain and brain stem are most common.
- Venous sinus thrombosis is common in Behcet's disease.

Further Reading

Chajek T, Fainaru M. Behçet's disease. Report of 41 cases and a review of the literature. *Medicine 54*:179–196, 1975.

Al Kawi MZ, Bohlega S, Banna M. MRI findings in neuro-Behçet's disease. *Neurology 41*:405–408, 1991.

Fasano A, D'Agostino M, Caldarola G, Feliciani C, De Simone C. Infliximab monotherapy in neuro-Behçet's disease: four year follow-up in a long-standing case resistant to conventional therapies. *J Neuroimmunol 239*:105–107, 2011.

32 CNS Sarcoidosis

A 45-year-old plastic surgeon is hospitalized for evaluation of progressive loss of vision in both eyes over the past 6 months. One month ago, he stopped operating. He is in good general health and has normal energy. He denies headache, seizures, nausea, tinnitus, hearing loss, trouble with speech or swallowing, focal paresthesias, weakness, or difficulty with balance. He is not taking any medications and was not exposed to any unusual chemicals or toxic materials. Mental status is normal. Visual acuity is 20/100 bilaterally. Visual fields are intact. Funduscopic examination reveals bilateral optic atrophy. Pupils are 6 mm in size and react sluggishly and incompletely to light. Extraocular movements are complete. The remainder of the cranial nerves, motor, sensory, coordination, and reflexes are normal. CBC, sedimentation rate, and renal and liver function studies are normal. The CSF opening pressure is normal. The CSF is clear and contains 118 WBCs, 98 percent mononuclear. CSF protein is 52 mg percent, and glucose is 60 mg percent. CSF gram stain, stain for acid-fast bacilli, VDRL, cryptococcal antigen, Lyme titer, and angiotensin-converting enzyme (ACE) levels are negative. Brain MRI reveals a nonenhancing mass infiltrating the optic chiasm.

What do you do now?

The patient's severely impaired visual acuity combined with an infiltrative legion in the optic chiasm would most likely be due to a glioma or, less likely, lymphoma. However the CSF pleocytosis indicates a chronic inflammatory disorder, most likely granulomatous disease (tuberculous or fungal meningitis, neurosyphilis, Lyme disease, or sarcoidosis). The acid-fast stain and culture of the CSF for bacteria and fungi, serologic test for syphilis, test for cryptococcal antigen, and serum and CSF ACE levels were all negative. No definitive diagnosis was possible initially, and he was treated empirically for tuberculous meningitis. Unfortunately, his vision continued to deteriorate and the CSF pleocytosis persisted. Because he was nearly blind, he was treated for 6 weeks with antifungal therapy, during which time his vision worsened to 20/400 and his CSF pleocytosis increased. To obtain a definitive diagnosis, a biopsy of the optic chiasm was performed. Pathologic examination revealed noncaseating granulomas, indicating CNS sarcoidosis. He was treated aggressively with high-dose steroids, but he developed diabetes insipidus and panhypopituitarism in the ensuing months and died.

Sarcoidosis is a multisystem granulomatous disorder of unknown etiology. Any organ may be affected, although the favored ones are lung, liver, lymph nodes, skin, bone, eyes, and salivary glands. Approximately 15 percent of all cases are pure CNS sarcoidosis. The neurologic manifestations of sarcoidosis are protean. Chronic meningitis with or without infarction is most common and frequently produces cranial nerve palsies. The optic, facial, and auditory nerves are particularly vulnerable. Sarcoidosis is among the few conditions that produce bilateral peripheral facial weakness (the others are lymphoma, Lyme disease, the Guillain-Barré syndrome and the Melkersson-Rosenthal syndrome). Diabetes insipidus in a patient with chronic meningitis strongly suggests CNS sarcoidosis. MRI scanning may reveal leptomeningeal enhancement or space-occupying lesions produced by CNS granulomas. Occasionally, disease is localized exclusively in white matter, mimicking lymphoma or multiple sclerosis. Sarcoid neuropathy or myopathy may also develop in the absence of systemic or CNS sarcoidosis. The CSF often contains hundreds to a few thousand WBCs, predominately mononuclear, elevated CSF protein, rarely a low CSF glucose, and sometimes increased IgG and oligoclonal bands. Elevated ACE levels are seen, but remember that increased ACE levels are also found in other infections and malignancy. The normal ACE levels in the patient may reflect the absence of widespread disease early in the clinical course. Histological diagnosis is generally confirmed by biopsy of lymph nodes, salivary glands, conjunctiva, skin, or liver. Meningeal or brain biopsy is a last resort. Treatment with corticosteroids often reduces the size of granulomas, but response to therapy is unpredictable. Patients who fail steroids have been given adjunctive immunosuppressive treatments including azathioprine, methotrexate, cyclophosphamide, cyclosporine, TNFα, pentoxifylline, thalidomide, etanercept, infliximab, and irradiation. The use of so many treatment modalities for one disease indicates the unpredictable response and lack of effectiveness of any single agent.

KEY POINTS TO REMEMBER

- Exclusive CNS disease accounts for 15 percent of all sarcoidosis.
- Sarcoidosis commonly presents as chronic meningitis with or without cerebral infarction.
- Cranial nerves II, VII, and VIII and the hypothalamus are particularly vulnerable in sarcoidosis.

Further Reading

Smith JK, Matheus MG, Castillo M. Imaging manifestations of neurosarcoidosis. *AJR Am J Roentgenol* 182:289-295, 2004.
Stern BJ. Neurological complications of sarcoidosis. *Curr Opin Neurol* 17:311-316, 2004.

33 Giant Cell (Temporal) Arteritis

An 81-year-old woman develops acute excruciating pain over the left side of her scalp. In recent weeks, she suspects low-grade fever, has loss of appetite, and is easily fatigued. She comments that chewing produces jaw pain. She denies any problems with cognition, vision, hearing, speech, balance, or focal weakness. Examination reveals nodularity and tenderness over the scalp above the ear. There is no history of muscle pain. The remainder of the neurologic examination, including her fundi, is normal. A blood count reveals mild anemia. Sedimentation rate is 45 mm/hour, and C-reactive protein (CRP) is 15μg/ml.

What do you do now?

The leading diagnosis must be giant cell (temporal) arteritis (GCA). Characteristic features include "headache" which, on careful questioning, often reveals that the patient is experiencing superficial pain over the scalp. Some patients will have TIAs or even stroke. Blindness occurs in GCA and is one reason that steroid therapy must be instituted promptly. Both the sedimentation rate and CRP are often elevated in GCA, and CRP increases are more common. Disease may extend beyond the cerebral arteries to involve the aorta. A history of polymyalgia rheumatica is seen in more than half of all patients with GCA. The primary pathologic change is necrosis in the arterial media (Fig. 33-1), often with multinucleated giant cells. GCA is treated with high-dose corticosteroids (e.g., prednisone, 1 mg/kg body weight) for 2–3 months before tapering. Treatment for 2–3 years is often necessary.

Importantly, varicella zoster virus (VZV) vasculopathy also causes scalp pain and visual loss, and is associated with a high sedimentation rate and elevated CRP. The pathology differs from that in GCA since early inflammation without necrosis is found in the arterial adventitia in VZV disease. GCA-negative temporal artery biopsy specimens should be examined for VZV antigen, particularly since the latter is amenable to treatment with antiviral therapy and can worsen with steroids alone.

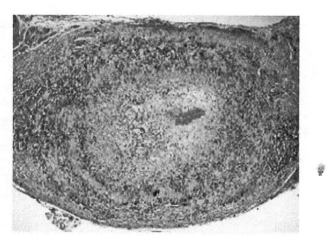

FIGURE 33-1 Temporal artery biopsy in giant cell (temporal) arteritis shows extensive inflammation and necrosis in arterial media.

- Fever occurs in less than half of patients with GCA and is usually low-grade.
- Headache is the most common symptom of GCA and occurs in 80–90 percent of patients; other symptoms include malaise, fatigue, anorexia, and weight loss, and are almost as common as headache.
- The most common sign of GCA is a nodular superficial temporal artery.
- GCA and polymyalgia rheumatica are part of a single disease spectrum.
- In GCA, CRP is elevated more often than the sedimentation rate.
- Temporal artery biopsy is positive in less than 50 percent of GCA.
- Treatment of GCA requires high-dose corticosteroids for 2–3 months before tapering.
- Because VZV vasculopathy, even without rash, also causes scalp pain and visual loss and is associated with a high sedimentation rate and elevated CRP, this diagnosis must also be considered in elderly patients with headache or periorbital pain and ischemic optic neuropathy with elevated CRP or sedimentation rates; GCA-negative temporal artery biopsy specimens should be examined for VZV antigen, particularly since VZV disease is amenable to treatment with antiviral therapy and can worsen with steroids alone.

Further Reading

Weyand CM, Goronzy JJ. Medium- and large-vessel vasculitis. *NEJM* 10;*349*:160–169, 2003.

Salazar R, Russman AN, Nagel MA, Cohrs RJ, Mahalingam R, Schmid DS, Kleinschmidt-DeMasters BK, VanEgmond EM, Gilden D. VZV ischemic optic neuropathy and subclinical temporal artery involvement. *Arch Neurol* 68:517–520, 2011.

Nagel MA , Russman AN, Feit H, Traktinskiy I, Khmeleva N, Schmid DS, Skarf B, Gilden D. VZV ischemic optic neuropathy and subclinical temporal artery infection without rash. *Neurology* 2013, In press.

Melkersson-Rosenthal
Syndrome

An 18-year-old man presents with swelling of his face
and lips. He reports three previous episodes of facial
paralysis on either side since childhood. Examination
reveals marked swelling of his entire face with peripheral
facial weakness bilaterally (Fig. 34-1). He reports that his
father also had intermittent episodes of facial weakness
and swelling. Examination of his tongue reveals deep
furrowing (Fig. 34-2) but no other abnormalities.

What do you do now?

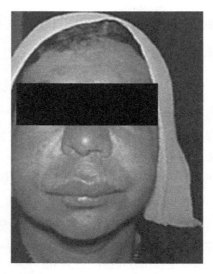

FIGURE 34-1 Melkersson-Rosenthal syndrome. Note swelling of the face and lips.

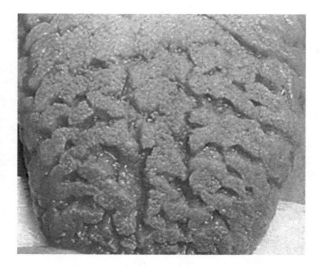

FIGURE 34-2 Melkersson-Rosenthal syndrome. Note deep (other clinical descriptors include plicated, scrotal, or geographic) furrowing of the tongue.

The triad of recurrent facial paralysis, facial edema, and a deeply furrowed (also known as geographic, scrotal, or plicated) tongue constitutes the Melkersson-Rosenthal syndrome. The condition is rare. Women are affected three times as often as men. The cause and pathogenesis of this syndrome are unknown. Biopsy of skin tissue reveals perivascular infiltrates of lymphocytes, plasma cells, and histiocytes as well as granulomas and multinucleated giant cells. Steroids have been used to reduce the inflammatory response. The effectiveness of surgery to release pressure on the facial nerves has not been established. Importantly, many people have deep fissuring of the tongue with no history of facial swelling or palsy. Melkersson-Rosenthal syndrome should be included in the differential diagnosis of recurrent facial palsy, which can also be seen in Lyme disease, sarcoidosis, and lymphoma.

KEY POINTS TO REMEMBER

- Melkersson-Rosenthal syndrome is characterized by the triad of recurrent facial paralysis, facial swelling, and a deeply fissured tongue.
- Melkersson-Rosenthal syndrome is a rare cause of recurrent peripheral facial palsy; other causes are Lyme disease, sarcoidosis, and lymphoma.
- Many people have a deeply fissured tongue with no history of facial swelling or weakness.

Further Reading

Greene RM, Rogers RS, 3rd. Melkersson-Rosenthal syndrome: a review of 36 patients. *J Am Acad Dermatol 21*:1263-1270, 1989.

Orlando MR, Atkins JS, Jr. Melkersson-Rosenthal Syndrome. *Arch Otolaryngol Head Neck Surg 116*:728-729, 1990.

English JB, Stommel EW, Bernat JL. Recurrent Bell's Palsy. *Neurology 47*:604-605, 1996.

35 Vogt-Koyanagi-Harada Syndrome (Uveomeningoencephalitis)

A 21-year-old Mexican American man presents with progressive loss of vision in both eyes and headache of 5 weeks' duration, mild fever, and neck pain. His initial visual problems began with blurriness in both eyes that gradually progressed to visual loss. In the past 3 weeks, he has noted ringing in both ears and intermittent periods of slurred speech. Examination reveals patchy bilateral periorbital vitiligo and diffuse alopecia over the scalp (Fig. 35-1). Visual acuity is 20/200 bilaterally. Both pupils are round, but react sluggishly to light. Funduscopic examination reveals bilateral retinal detachments. Slit lamp examination discloses inflammatory cells in the vitreous and uveal tract. There is horizontal nystagmus with a rotary component bilaterally, greater when looking to the left. Air conduction is reduced in both ears, more so on the right. The Weber test localizes to the left side. The remainder of the cranial nerves, motor examination, and coordination are normal. There is a moderate gait ataxia. DTRs are normal, and both plantar responses are flexor. A brain MRI is normal. The CSF opening pressure is normal. The CSF is clear and contains 85 WBCs, all mononuclear; CSF protein is 52 mg percent, glucose is normal, no oligoclonal bands are detected, and cytology is negative. An ophthalmology consultant notes bilateral chorioretinal folds and serous retinal detachments and edema in both maculae, as confirmed by optical coherence tomography (Fig. 35-2). Sedimentation rate and angiotensin-converting enzyme levels are normal, and VDRL is negative.

What do you do now?

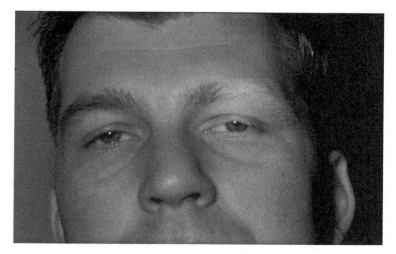

FIGURE 35-1 Vogt-Koyanagi-Harada syndrome. Patchy orbital vitiligo over the eyelids and alopecia over the scalp.

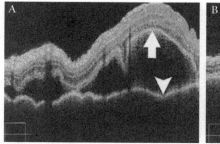 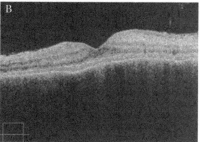

FIGURE 35-2 Optical coherence tomography shows serous retinal detachment and edema (A) that resolved after steroid treatment (B). (From Loh Y. Basilar leptomeningitis in Vogt-Koyanagi-Harada disease. *Neurology* 78(6):438-439; 2012. Reprinted with permission from Wolters Kluwer Health.)

The patient has a subacute progressive illness characterized by uveitis, meningeal inflammation, and CNS disease. Infectious agents that cause a uveomeningeal syndrome include tuberculosis, syphilis, toxoplasmosis, fungi, and several viruses such as cytomegalovirus, herpes simplex virus, and varicella zoster virus. A uveomeningeal syndrome may also occur in sarcoidosis, Wegener's granulomatosis, and Behcet's disease. The presence of ocular and neurologic disease in a patient with pigmentary changes and vitiligo around the eye and on the scalp is characteristic of uveomeningoencephalitis known as the Vogt-Koyanagi-Harada syndrome. The organ most severely affected is the eye, in which inflammation of the uveal tract (uveitis) predominates. Patients present with decreased vision and floaters. Funduscopic examination reveals white sheathing of retinal vessels, an indication of retinal vasculitis. Inflammatory cells are also present in the vitreous humor. Retinal detachment is common. Neurologic disease may present at the time of uveitis or months later. Neurologic complications are protean and include headache, stiff neck, seizures, and focal deficit. Tinnitus, hearing loss, and vertigo are frequent. A mononuclear CSF pleocytosis is characteristic. The pathogenesis of Vogt-Koyanagi-Harada syndrome is not well understood, but may reflect a T-cell-mediated autoimmune response against melanocyte antigen. T cells from patients with disease who have HLA-DRB1–0405 display a peptide-specific Th1 response when sensitized to melanocyte epitopes. Indirect but tantalizing evidence that a virus triggers disease is based on the observation that focal loss of pigmentation along vascular channels in skin is strikingly similar to the "color break" seen in virus-infected tulips (Fig. 35-3). Treatment usually begins with systemic steroids; in refractory cases, multiple cytotoxic drugs have been used.

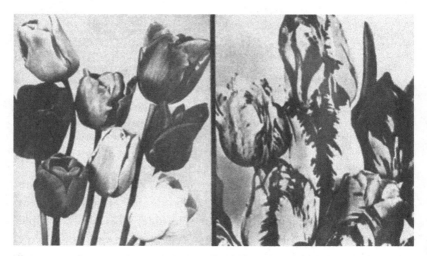

FIGURE 35-3 Note healthy tulips (left) compared to "Rembrandt" tulips (right) that exhibit a virus-induced "color break." (From Nelhaus G. Acquired unilateral vitiligo and poliosis of the head and subacute encephalitis with partial recovery. *Neurology 20*(10):965-974; 1970. Reprinted with permission from Wolters Kluwer Health.)

- In patients with ocular and neurological disease, look carefully at the skin around the eyes and scalp for patchy vitiligo and hair loss.

Further Reading

Inomata H, Kato M. Vogt-Koyanagi-Harada disease. In: *Handbook of Clinical Neurology* (Vinken PJ, Bruyn GW, Klawans HL, McKendall RR, eds). Amsterdam: Elsevier Science, Vol. 12, 611–626, 1989.

Damico FM, Cunha-Neto E, Goldberg AC, Iwai LK, Marin ML, Hammer J, Kalil J, Yamamoto JH. T-cell recognition and cytokine profile induced by melanocyte epitopes in patients with HLA-DRB1*0405-positive and -negative Vogt-Koyanagi-Harada uveitis. *Invest Ophthalmol Vis Sci 46*:2465–2471, 2005.

Index